Anae
at the district hospital

Michael B. Dobson

Consultant Anaesthetist
Nuffield Department of Anaesthetics
John Radcliffe Hospital
Oxford
England

illustrated by
Derek Atherton
and Elisabetta Sacco

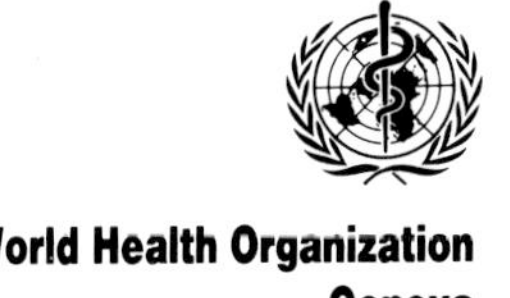

World Health Organization
Geneva
1988

Reprinted 1991, 1993

ISBN 92 4 154228 4

Printed in Switzerland
87/7456 — Atar — 7500
91/8858 — Atar — 3000 (R)
93/9680 — Atar — 3000

CONTENTS

Preface

This handbook is one of three[1] to be published by the World Health Organization for the guidance of doctors providing surgical and anaesthetic services in small district hospitals (hospitals of first referral) with limited access to specialist services. The advice offered has been deliberately restricted to procedures that may need to be carried out by a young doctor with limited experience in anaesthesia, surgery, or obstetrics, using the facilities that can reasonably be expected in such hospitals. Wherever possible, the drugs, equipment, and radiodiagnostic and laboratory procedures described conform with WHO and UNICEF recommendations.

Although the handbooks contain detailed descriptions and illustrations, the advice they offer is no substitute for practical experience. The reader is expected to have been exposed to all the relevant techniques during undergraduate or early postgraduate education. When necessary the text indicates which patients should be referred for specialized care at a higher level, as it is important to developing health services that young doctors and their superiors understand the limitations of practice at the district hospital.

It has, of course, been necessary to be selective in deciding what to include in the handbooks, but it is hoped that any important omissions will be revealed during field testing. WHO would also be pleased to receive comments and suggestions regarding the handbooks and experience with their use. Such comments would be of considerable value in the preparation of any future editions of the books. Finally, it is hoped that the handbooks will fulfil their purpose — to help doctors working at the front line of surgery throughout the world.

The three handbooks have been prepared in collaboration with the following organizations:

- Christian Medical Commission
- International College of Surgeons
- International Council of Nurses
- International Federation of Gynaecology and Obstetrics
- International Federation of Surgical Colleges
- International Society of Burn Injuries
- International Society of Orthopaedic Surgery and Traumatology
- League of Red Cross and Red Crescent Societies
- World Federation of Societies of Anaesthesiologists
- World Orthopaedic Concern.

Acknowledgements

This handbook has been prepared as part of a collaborative activity between WHO and the World Federation of Societies of Anaesthesiologists, which reviewed and endorsed the draft manuscript and illustrations. In this regard, the support of Dr John Zorab, WFSA Secretary, is gratefully acknowledged.

[1] Also in preparation: *General surgery at the district hospital* and *Surgery at the district hospital: obstetrics, gynaecology, orthopaedics, and traumatology.*

1 Introduction

This volume has been produced to help medical officers in small hospitals to provide safe and effective anaesthesia for their patients. Because the resources available for health care are limited, especially in these small hospitals, many anaesthetic services are subject to constraints on personnel, equipment, and drugs. An anaesthetic service must therefore strike a balance that meets most clinical needs most of the time, rather than strive for perfection in some areas while neglecting others. Difficulty in obtaining sufficient supplies, particularly of items that must be imported, may mean that there are no reserves of drugs or spare equipment in the hospital. Anaesthetic techniques for such a hospital should therefore depend as little as possible on external supplies and technology (equipment, expertise for maintenance work, etc.). The needs of a small hospital are best served by the regular use of relatively few anaesthetic techniques that can provide good anaesthesia for virtually any clinical situation. This book is intended to be a manual of such techniques.

Anaesthesia is now much safer and more pleasant for the patient than it was 50 years ago. Factors contributing to the improvements include a fuller understanding of physiology and pharmacology; better preoperative assessment and preparation of patients; closer monitoring of anaesthetized patients; and the introduction of new techniques, such as the use of muscle relaxants, endotracheal intubation, and calibrated vaporizers for volatile anaesthetic agents. Improvements in anaesthesia have allowed surgeons to attempt more complicated operations on increasing numbers of patients, and this has resulted in a growing demand for and a shortage of anaesthetists. In many small hospitals a specialist anaesthetist will not be available, and anaesthesia will be the responsibility of a medical officer with one or two years of postgraduate training, who will need to provide anaesthesia not only for routine elective surgery but also for emergency surgery requiring more major procedures, when a life-threatening condition prevents referral of the patient to a larger hospital. A medical officer who is thoroughly familiar with a small clinical repertoire of safe anaesthetic techniques will be well equipped to deal with both elective and emergency cases.

Every anaesthetist needs a foundation of basic medical science for his or her clinical techniques. A sound knowledge of physiology and pharmacology is essential, together with an understanding of the changes brought about by illness or injury. However, these subjects are normally dealt with during undergraduate training and are beyond the scope of this short book.

Many techniques originally developed for use during anaesthesia are now widely recognized as applicable to the care of a variety of critically ill patients, for example those with severe head injuries, asthma, tetanus, or neonatal asphyxia. Skills such as the rapid assessment and management of unconscious patients, control of the airway, endotracheal intubation, management of the circulation, and cardiopulmonary resuscitation have their origins in anaesthesia, but are now recognized as essential for all doctors.

Good anaesthesia depends much more on the skills, training, and standards of the anaesthetist than on the availability of expensive and complicated equipment. Even if it is difficult to obtain medical gases, a small hospital must still provide an anaesthetic service. This can be achieved by the use of draw-over anaesthetic techniques, in which ambient air is used as the carrier gas to which volatile anaesthetic agents are added by calibrated, low-resistance vaporizers. If oxygen is available, it can be used to enrich the inspired gas mixture, but it is not essential; nitrous oxide, which is harder to obtain and more expensive than oxygen, is unnecessary. Draw-over techniques are capable of producing first-class clinical anaesthesia; the apparatus is simple to understand and use, and can usually be serviced locally. Compared with systems dependent on compressed medical gases, draw-over systems are economical in use and have added safety in that the lowest oxygen concentration that can be delivered is that of air. Draw-over anaesthesia is the system of first choice for small hospitals; it should also be in regular use in larger and teaching hospitals as one of a range of techniques. Since some small hospitals are already equipped with continuous-flow (Boyle's) anaesthetic apparatus, its use is also covered in this manual. Continuous-flow machines require compressed medical gases for use, and great care is needed to avoid the accidental delivery of hypoxic gas mixtures to the patient. Techniques of conduction (local or regional) anaesthesia are also described here, though they are best learned from practical clinical teaching. It is a common mistake to believe that general anaesthesia is "dangerous" and conduction anaesthesia "safe". Conduction anaesthesia has a valuable and important place in anaesthesia, but requires the same care and attention to the preparation and selection of patients as does general anaesthesia, because serious adverse reactions can and do occur.

Anaesthesia is a practical clinical subject as well as an academic study. This manual alone cannot teach you to be a safe and skilled anaesthetist — no book could. A period of clinical teaching under the close supervision of an experienced anaesthetist is essential, both at the beginning of training and at regular intervals thereafter. Such training can be arranged either by attachment of medical officers to larger hospitals or by organizing regular visits by specialist anaesthetists to smaller hospitals. Experience can also be a good teacher, and the best way to make use of it is to keep a careful record of every anaesthetic given and to review these records with colleagues at regular intervals. No hospital is too small to benefit from regular clinical reviews and no doctor too wise to benefit from the experience of colleagues.

This is a limited book with limited aims. Readers who decide to become specialist anaesthetists will ultimately find its range of techniques too restrictive and will move on to more extensive textbooks, but the basic principles of safe anaesthesia set out here will continue to serve them well.

2
Fundamental techniques and skills

With the establishment of anaesthesia as a major medical speciality over the last 50 years, a number of anaesthesia-related skills have emerged. These skills were originally used primarily in the care and protection of anaesthetized patients, but they are now recognized as essential for all doctors who deal with unconscious or critically ill patients, and are particularly important for those working in small hospitals who may have to bear responsibility for all aspects of a patient's welfare and management. The range of such skills includes:

- assessment of the critically ill and/or unconscious patient
- care of the airway
- care of the patient whose breathing is inadequate
- management of the circulation
- assessment of the effects of treatment
- transportation of the critically ill patient.

Once acquired, these skills are relevant both to the immediate care of a variety of critically ill patients — for example, those with severe dehydration, head injury, or major blood loss — and to the proficient and safe practice of clinical anaesthesia.

Assessment of the critically ill and/or unconscious patient

To identify any immediate threat to life and start treatment, you must be able to make a brief and rapid assessment of a patient who is critically ill. In many cases the cause of the patient's condition is obvious, but it may help you to remember the letters A-B-C-B-A:

A — **A**irway
B — **B**reathing
C — **C**irculation
B — **B**rain
A — **A**ssess other injuries.

This initial assessment should take only a few moments:

A — Check whether the patient has a clear airway.
B — Check whether the patient is breathing; if not, he or she will need immediate artificial ventilation.
C — Check for pulsation in a major vessel (carotid or femoral arteries); if there is a circulatory arrest, start external cardiac massage immediately.
B — Assess the patient's brain function; note responses to speech, stimulation, or pain, and also pupillary size and any abnormal posture.
A — Rapidly assess any associated injuries, including "hidden" ones such

as a pneumothorax or pelvic fracture, and estimate the extent of blood loss or fluid depletion.

Once you have made your rapid assessment, you may decide that one or more aspects of the patient's condition demand priority. Their management is outlined below.

Care of the airway

Any severely injured or unconscious patient lying supine is in extreme danger of airway obstruction and asphyxiation. The tongue falls backwards in this position, causing partial or complete obstruction of the pharynx. Airway obstruction of this type is by far the commonest cause of preventable death after head injury. First check the mouth and pharynx for the presence of any foreign body. Once this is done, and provided that the patient is breathing and there is no contraindication to movement (such as suspected spinal injury), turn him or her over into the semiprone or coma position with the upper arm and leg flexed. If it is not possible to turn the patient, for example during anaesthesia, the airway may be kept clear by one of the following means.

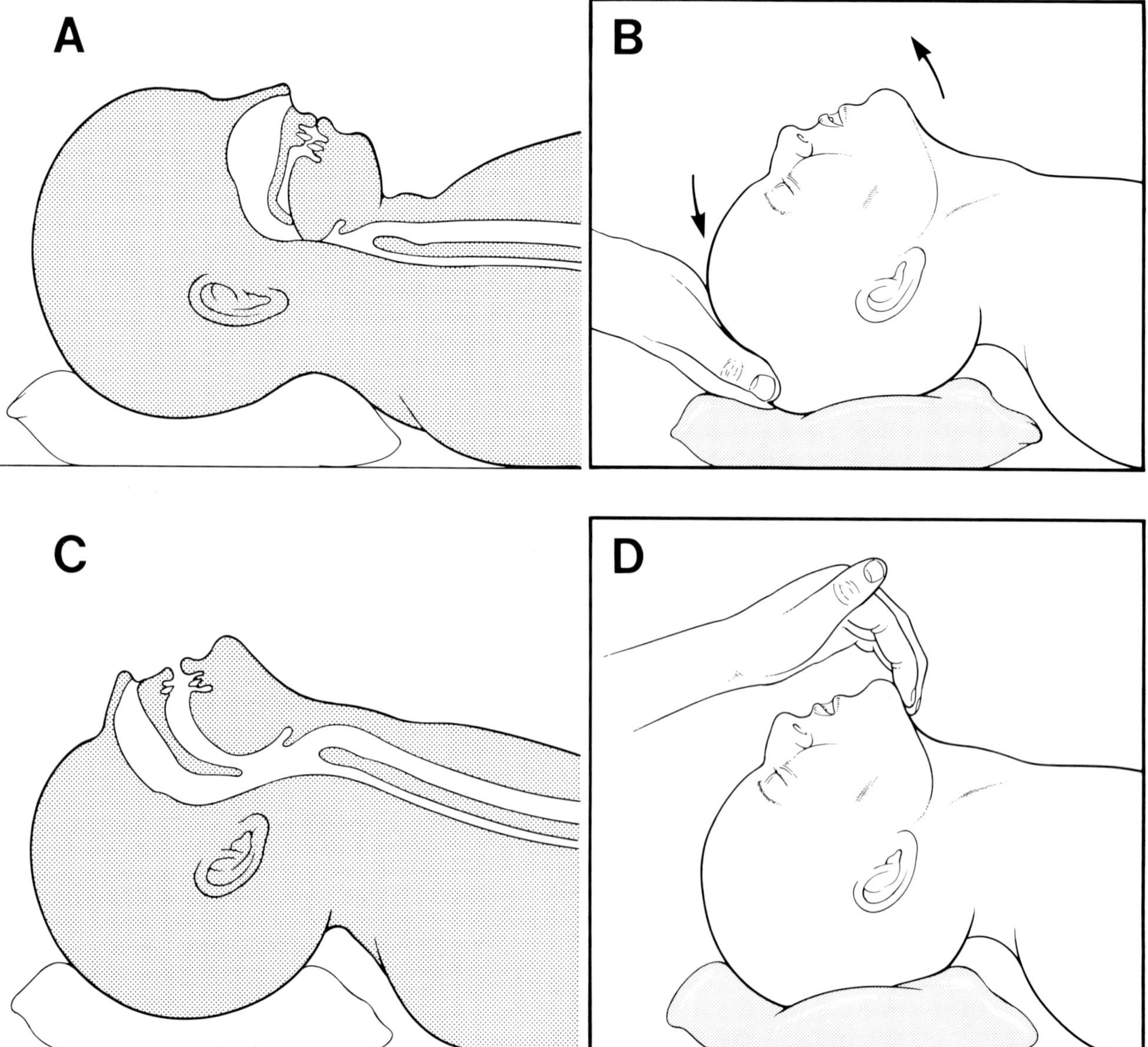

Fig. 2.1. Clearing the airway by extension of the head. (A) Mechanism of airway obstruction when supine; (B,C) extension of the head; (D) maintaining a clear airway by supporting the jaw.

Repositioning the head and neck

Extension of the head combined with forward displacement of the jaw (which lifts the tongue forward by its attachment to the jaw) will often clear the airway (Fig. 2.1). To keep the airway clear you will need to maintain traction, either by lifting the anterior part of the jaw or by pressing forwards and upwards with your thumbs at the angle of the jaw.

Inserting an artificial airway

An oropharyngeal or nasopharyngeal airway will help to maintain a clear air passage (Fig. 2.2 & 2.3). An oropharyngeal airway should be lubricated before insertion with lubricating gel or water, but never liquid paraffin (mineral oil). Insert it with the concave side facing upwards, and then rotate it into its final position as it enters the pharynx. In a patient with tightly clenched teeth, a nasopharyngeal airway is sometimes helpful; insert it gently to avoid causing a nosebleed. If a nasal airway is not available, insert an endotracheal tube through the nose until its tip lies just above the tip of the epiglottis. Do not use gags and wedges to force open a patient's mouth; they are damaging and potentially dangerous. A patient whose mouth is firmly closed can be managed either in the coma position if intubation is not possible or, preferably, by endotracheal intubation using a relaxant.

Endotracheal intubation

The insertion of an endotracheal tube provides a clear airway and protects the patient's lungs against the aspiration of gastric contents. Inserting an endotracheal tube is not particularly difficult, and every doctor should be capable of performing this life-saving manoeuvre. The technique is now widely taught to doctors, nurses, anaesthetic assistants, and ambulance crews, and once you have mastered it you should teach it to others also.

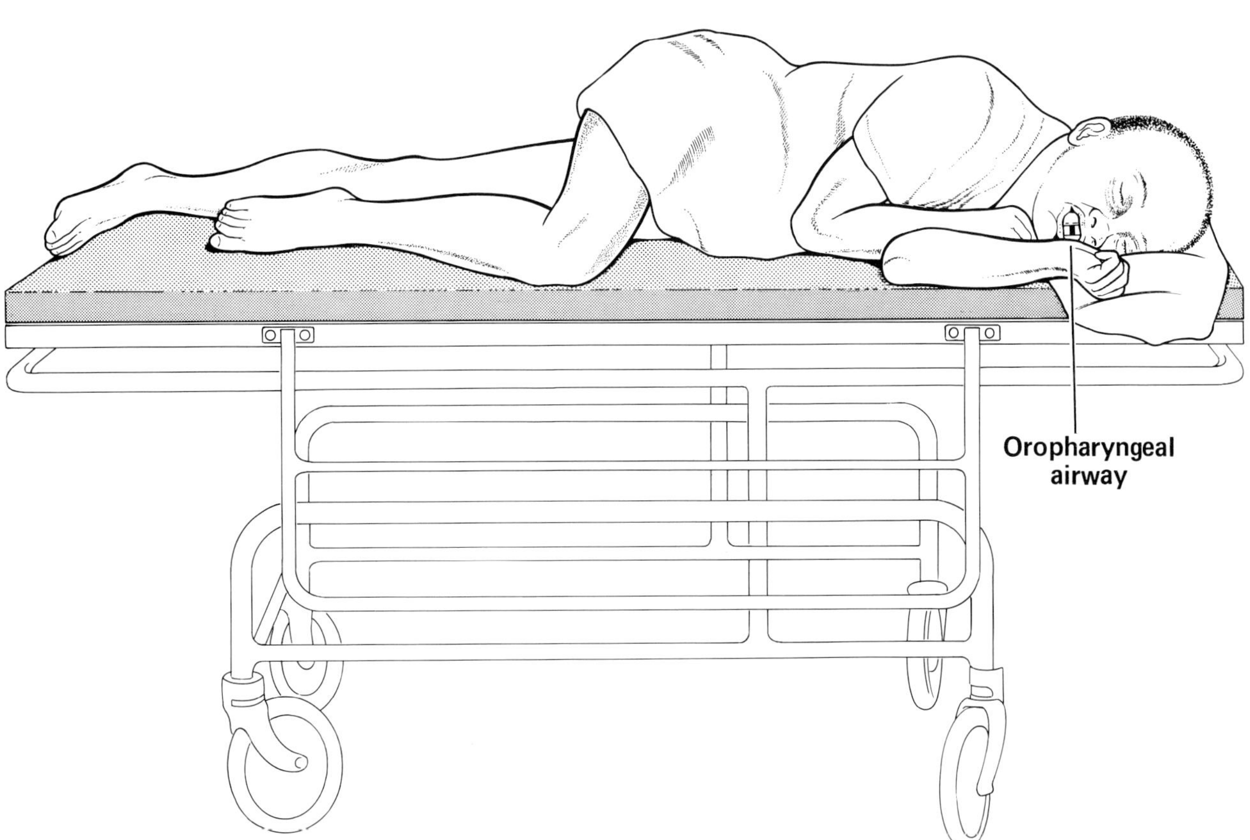

Fig. 2.2. The use of an oropharyngeal airway with the patient in the semiprone (coma) position.

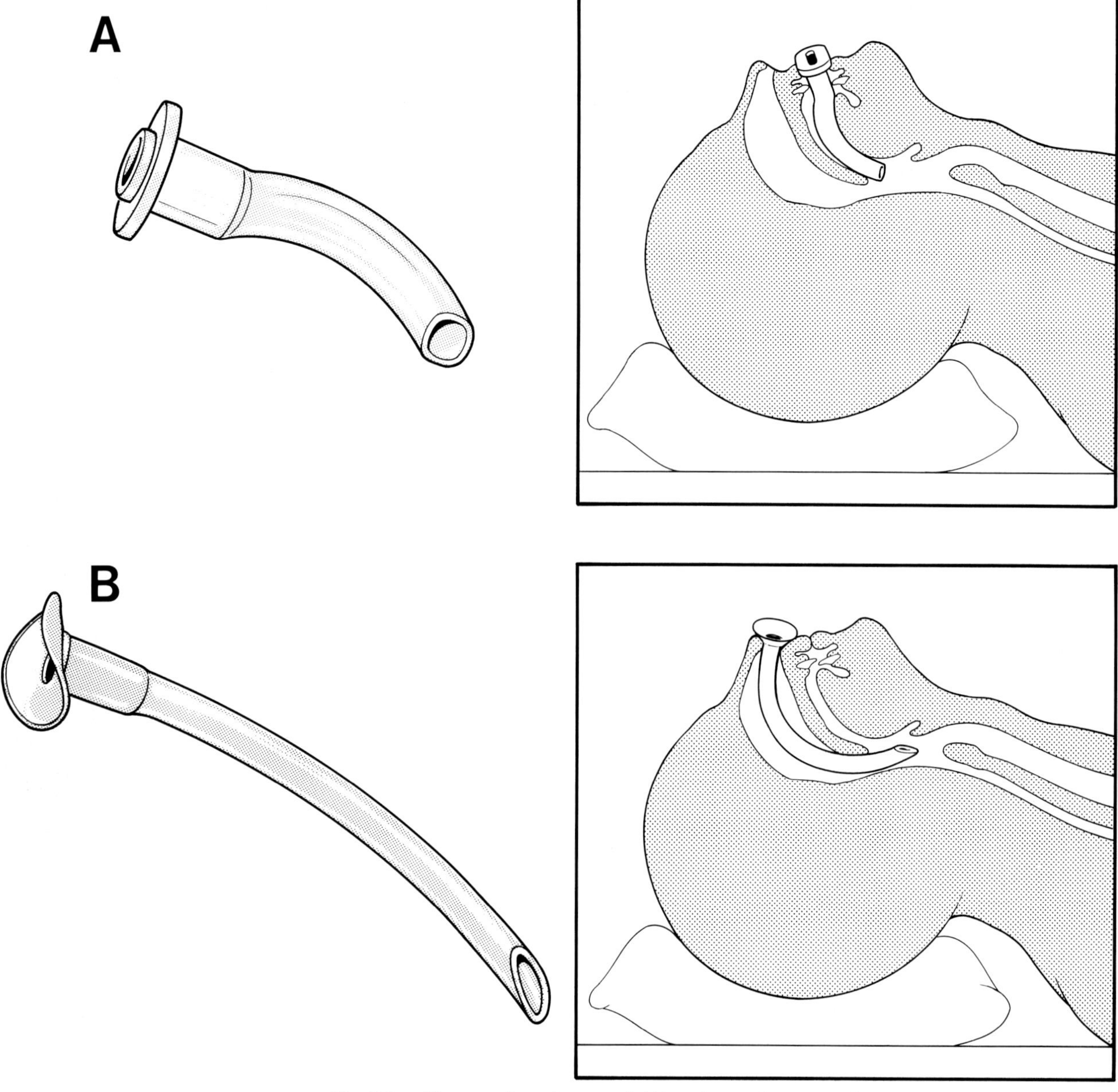

Fig. 2.3. The use of oropharyngeal (A) and nasopharyngeal (B) airways.

Endotracheal intubation can be performed in the following circumstances:

- conscious patients — suitable for neonates and certain adult emergencies
- unconscious patients — no preparation needed
- anaesthetized patients — light anaesthesia, with a relaxant
  — deep anaesthesia, without a relaxant.

If you are inexperienced, it is much safer to intubate without giving a relaxant, since if intubation fails the patient can still breathe.

Technique of endotracheal intubation

You will need a trained assistant and the following basic equipment (some of which is shown in Fig. 2.4):

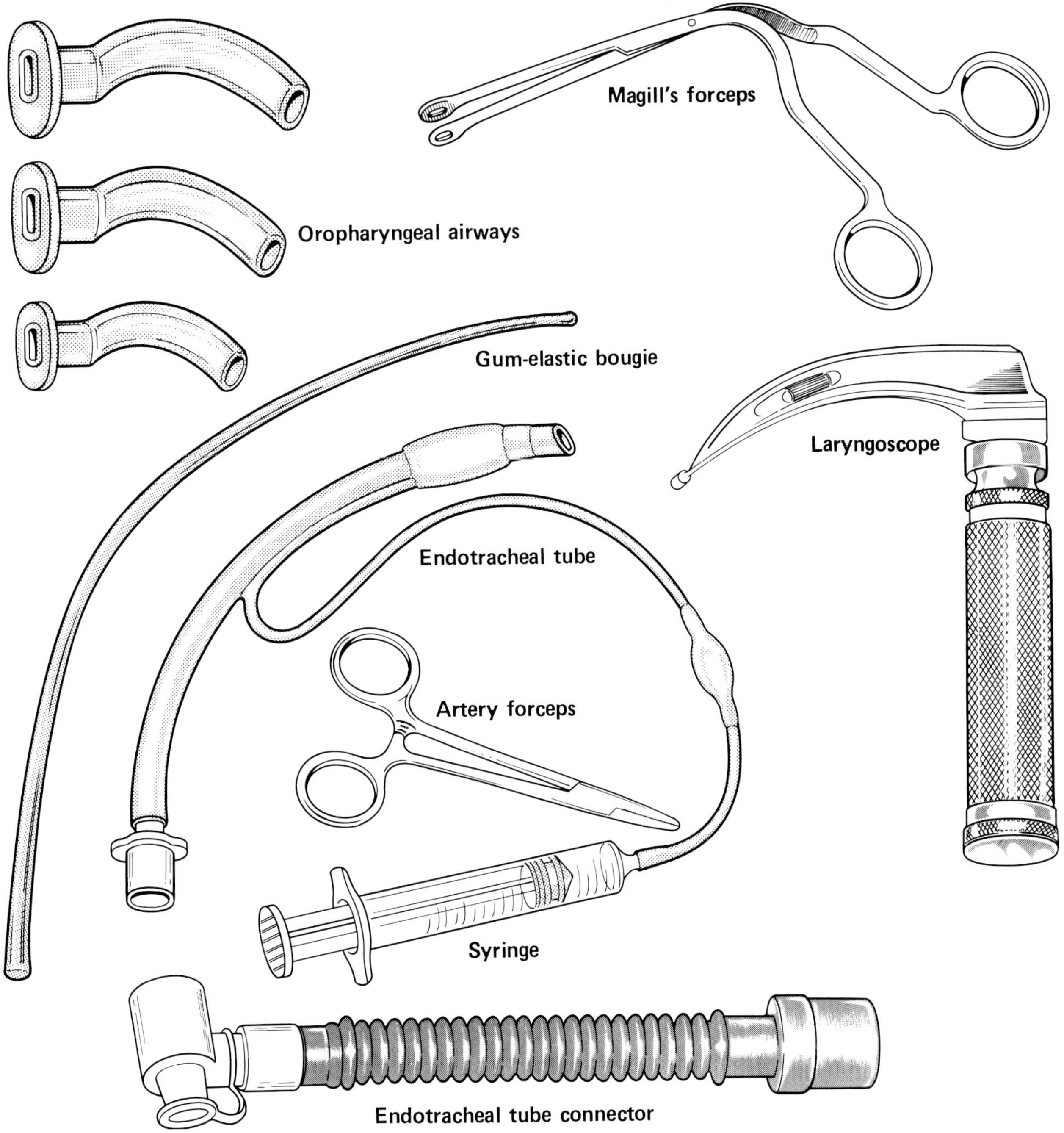

Fig. 2.4. Some of the equipment needed for endotracheal intubation.

- functioning laryngoscope and spare
- suitably sized endotracheal tube
- Magill's intubating forceps
- suction apparatus (electric or manual)
- anaesthetic face mask
- means of inflating the lungs with mask or tube, for example a self-inflating bag or bellows (SIB).

Position of the head and neck

The best possible view of the larynx is obtained by having the neck slightly flexed and the head extended on the neck. In most adults this can be achieved by placing one or even two pillows under the head; the different proportions of a child's body mean that for younger children no pillow is needed and that for the neonate it may be necessary to put a small pillow under the shoulders (Fig. 2.5).

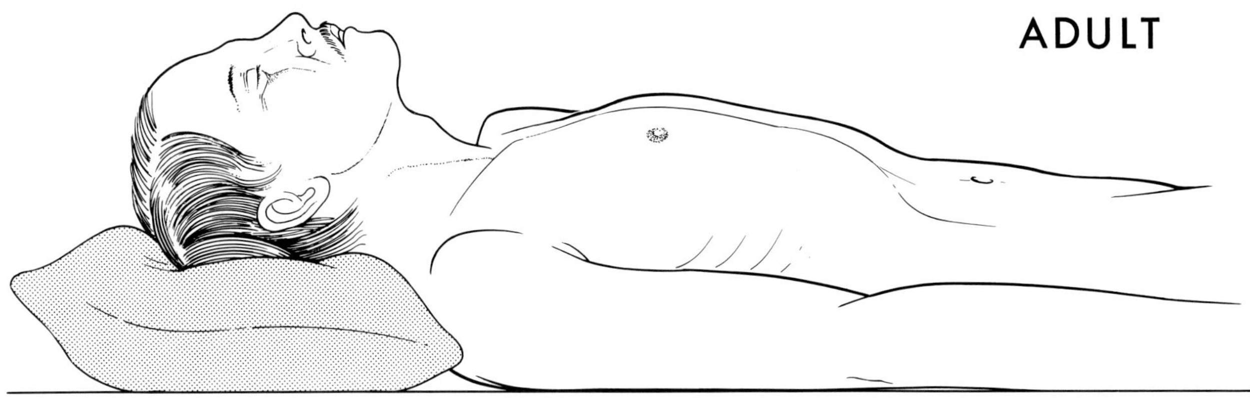

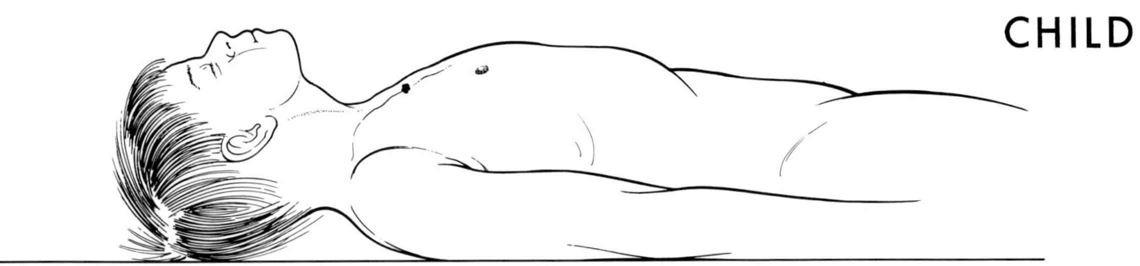

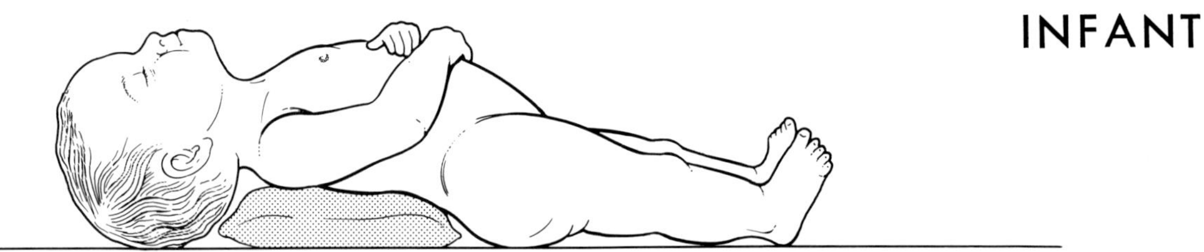

Fig. 2.5. Position of the head and neck for endotracheal intubation.

Oxygenation

Even if relaxants are not used, the patient's breathing during the process of intubation is likely to be impaired; you should therefore first give the patient oxygen from a closely fitting face mask (Fig. 2.6A) — 10 good breaths are enough. If the patient is not breathing, gently inflate the lungs using a face mask and an SIB. *Never* try to intubate a cyanosed patient without first inflating the lungs a few times with a face mask, even if only air is available.

Use of the laryngoscope

Take the laryngoscope in your left hand. Insert the blade gently into the right side of the patient's mouth and pass it back over the tongue until you can see the uvula (Fig. 2.6B–E). (By now the tip of the blade should be in the midline.) Advance the blade a little further, and the tip of the epiglottis will come into view; the blade should pass between the epiglottis and the base of the tongue (Fig. 2.6F,G). Lift the laryngoscope towards the ceiling (do not lever with the patient's front teeth as a fulcrum), and the laryngeal opening will be revealed below and behind the epiglottis, with the white vocal cords visible anteriorly and the arytenoid cartilages posteriorly (Fig. 2.6H–J).

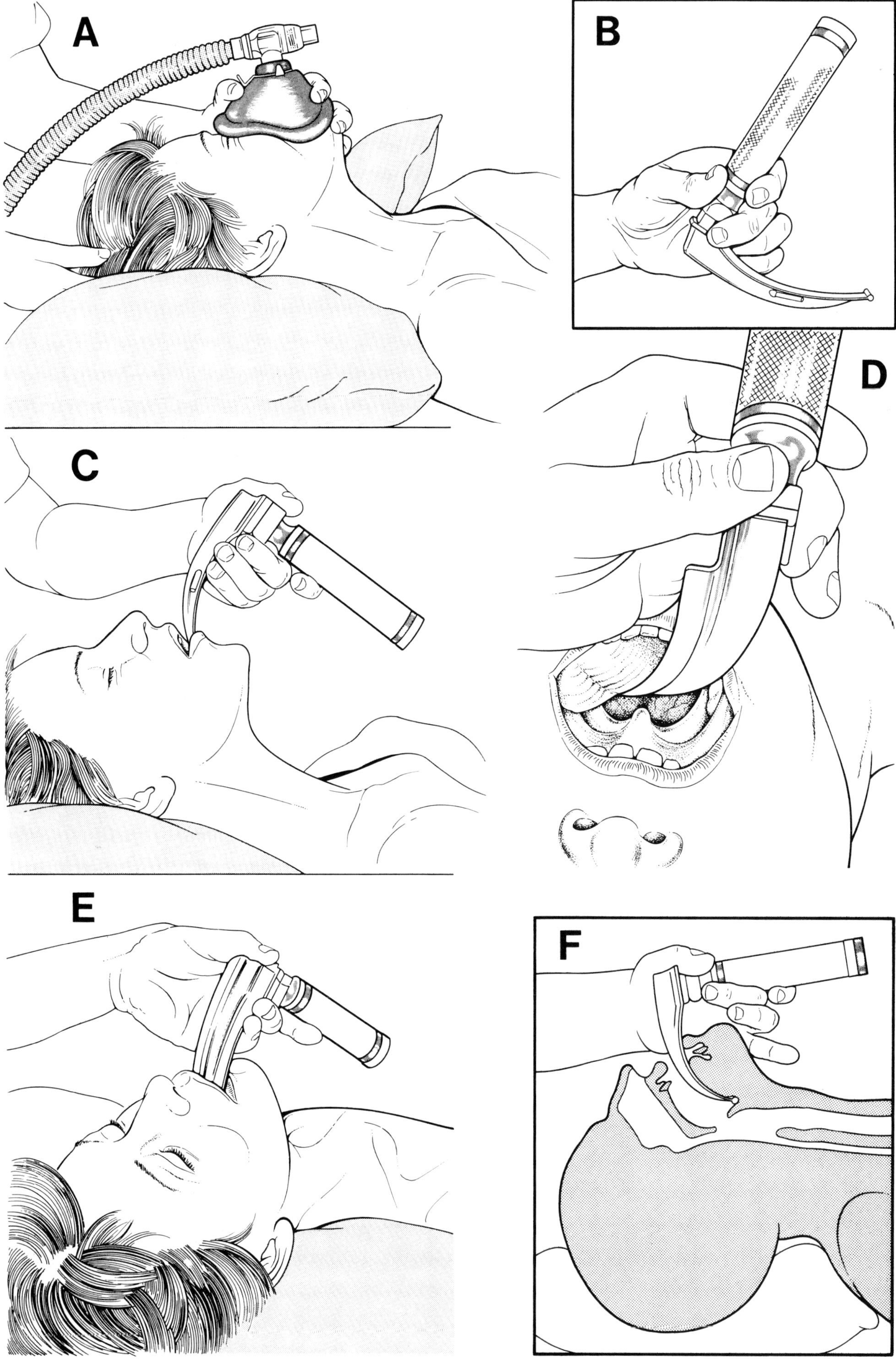

Fig. 2.6. Technique of endotracheal intubation. (A) Inflate the lungs with oxygen. (B) Take the laryngoscope with your left hand. (C) Insert the laryngoscope blade gently in the right side of the mouth. (D,E) Initial view of the oropharynx. (F) Insert the blade between the epiglottis and the base of the tongue.

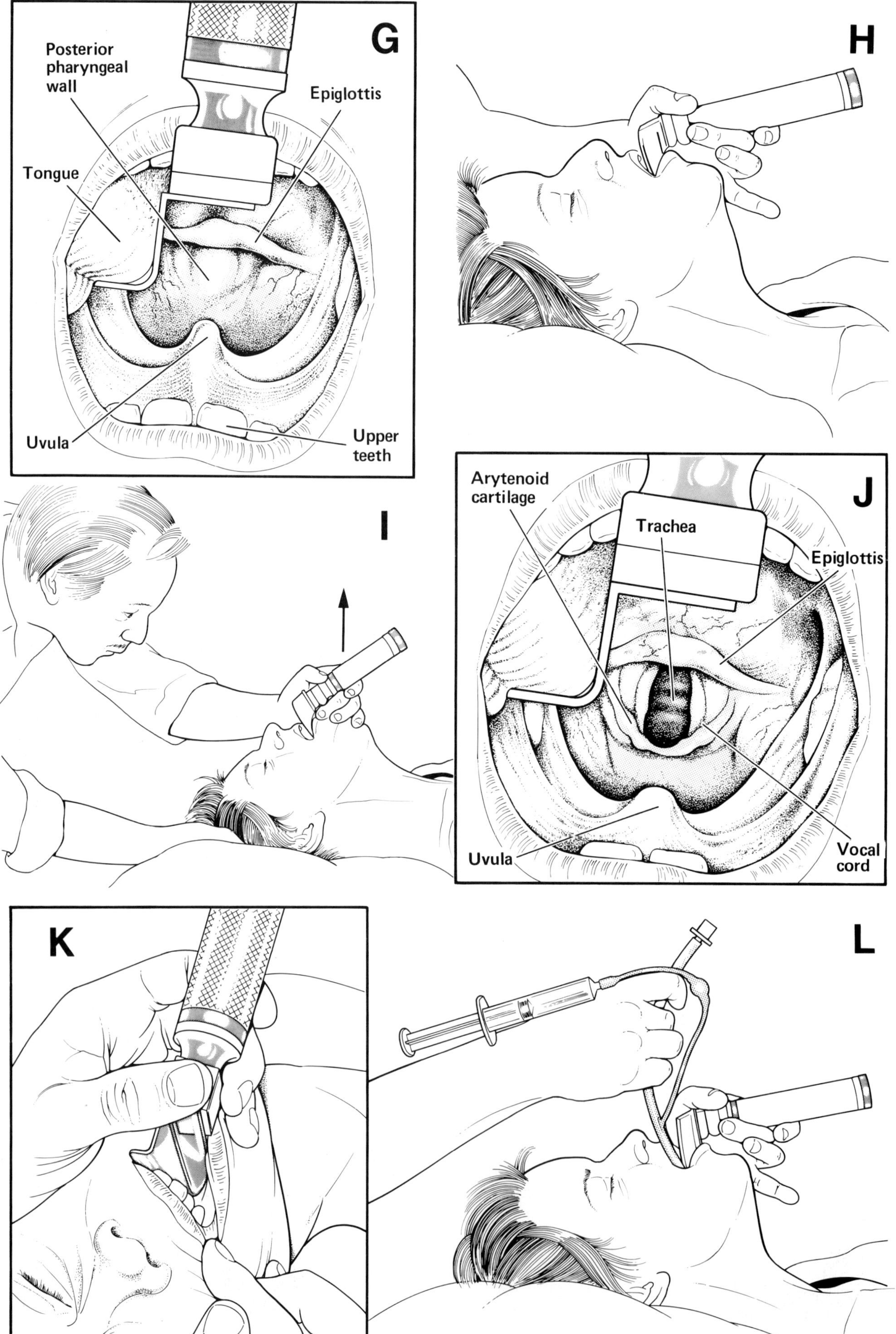

Fig. 2.6. Technique of endotracheal intubation *(continued)*. (G) View of the pharynx and epiglottis. (H,I) Lift the blade towards the ceiling. (J) View of the larynx. (K) Retract the lip to improve the view. (L) Insert the endotracheal tube.

Inserting the tube

Your assistant should now pass you the endotracheal tube; take it in your right hand and pass it carefully down through the mouth and pharynx (avoid touching the side walls if possible) and between the vocal cords. If you do not have a good view of the cords:

- Ask your assistant to press gently back on the thyroid cartilage; this should displace the larynx back into your field of vision.
- Your assistant should also retract the upper lip upwards to give you a clearer view (Fig. 2.6K).
- If you can see the arytenoid cartilages, but not the cords, pass the tube in the midline between these cartilages and the epiglottis, and it will usually enter the trachea (Fig. 2.6L). This may be easier if you pass a urethral bougie down the inside of the endotracheal tube, with 3–4 cm projecting distally and curved forwards (Fig. 2.6M). If using Oxford or armoured latex endotracheal tubes, you will always need a bougie.

Checking the position of the tube

After intubation it is essential to check the position of the endotracheal tube to ensure that it has passed neither into the oesophagus, nor into one of the main bronchi (which would cause collapse of the opposite lung). The best way to be sure that the tube is not in the oesophagus is to have seen it go into the larynx. Failing this, if the patient is breathing and you can feel breath and hear breath sounds at the top end of the tube, it is correctly placed; if the tube is in the oesophagus the patient will breathe around and not through it. If the patient is not breathing, for example after having been given a relaxant, give a sharp tap on the sternum; if the tube has entered the trachea, you should feel a small puff of air escape from the tube. Check by blowing air down the tube with an SIB; if the tube is correctly placed, the chest wall will rise and fall as air enters and leaves, but if the tube is in the oesophagus, there will be a gurgling sound and only the stomach will inflate. You should also check the position of the tube by listening with a stethoscope over each lung base and over the stomach while assisting ventilation manually. A further indication of correct intubation is that the non-paralysed patient will often cough if you pass a suction catheter down the endotracheal tube.

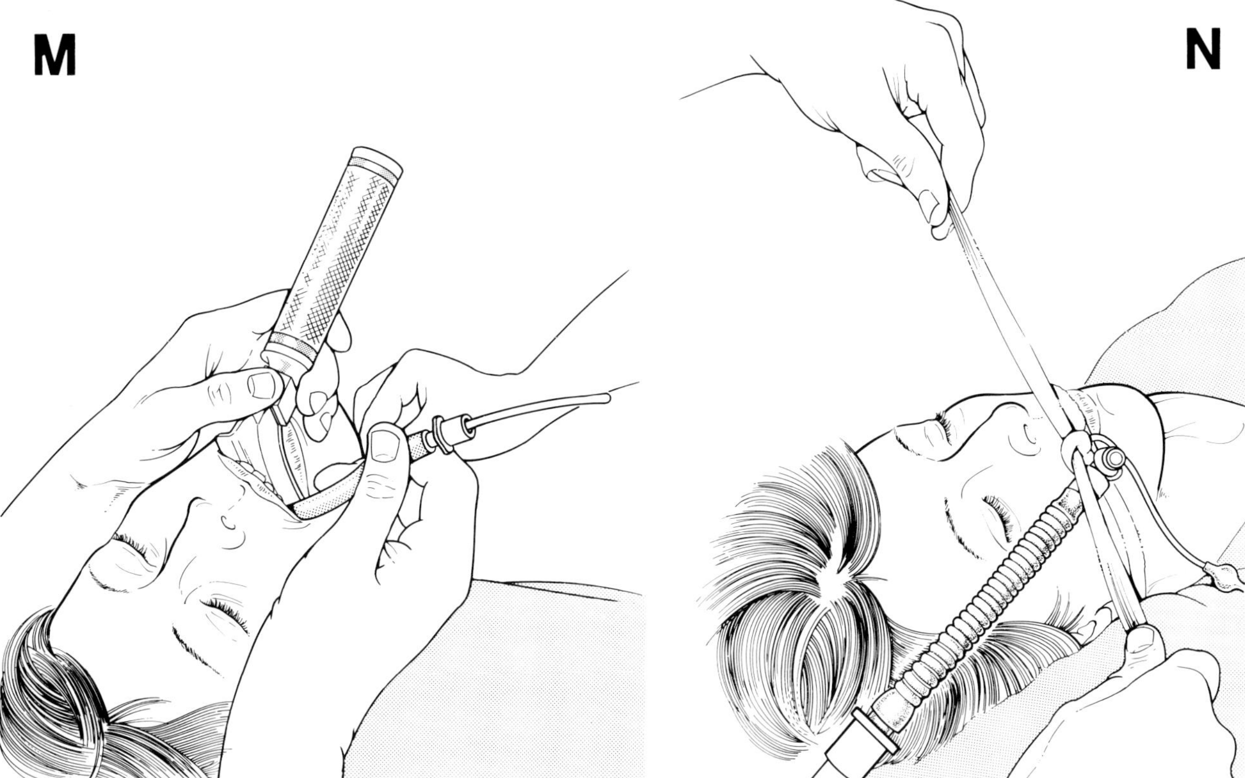

Fig. 2.6. Technique of endotracheal intubation *(continued)*. (M) Use a bougie to help direct the tube while your assistant applies cricoid pressure, if necessary. (N) Securely fix the tube in place.

Once you are sure the tube has entered the trachea, you must check that it has not gone too far and entered a main bronchus. To do this, inflate the lungs manually while listening in turn over both lung apices and both bases. Air entry should be equal on the two sides. If the tube is too far in, it will usually have entered the right main bronchus and there will be no air entry or chest wall movement on the left. If this is so, withdraw the tube 2–3 cm and listen again until air entry is uniform. Once you are certain that the endotracheal tube is correctly positioned, fix it securely in place (Fig. 2.6N).

Remember that it is much safer for an inexperienced person to intubate without giving the patient relaxants, since if intubation fails the patient can still breathe.

The golden rule of intubation

If at the end of the procedure you are not certain of the position of the tip of the tube, you must remove it and begin again.

Failed intubation

Every anaesthetist, no matter how experienced, has difficulty with intubation on occasion, although the occasions become rarer with increasing experience. You may have little time to spare before attempting emergency intubation of a severely injured or unconscious patient. However, if you are inserting an endotracheal tube for anaesthesia, you will be less likely to have an unpleasant surprise during intubation if you make a practice of specifically assessing the patient beforehand for features likely to hinder intubation. For example, check whether the patient has a receding jaw, awkward teeth, a restricted mouth opening, a stiff neck, or swellings in the neck. If you decide that intubation will be difficult, and anaesthesia is necessary, use an inhalational induction and intubation technique. Although slower than an intravenous technique, it is much safer. The worst problems are always the ones you have not anticipated.

If you have just had one unsuccessful attempt at intubation, proceed as follows. First make sure that the patient is oxygenated by inflating the lungs with the bag/bellows and face mask. If you cannot do this, there must be:

- an obstruction in the airway,
- laryngeal spasm, or
- a leak around the face mask.

If you cannot rapidly correct the problem, you must oxygenate the patient quickly by another method. Insert a large (14-gauge or, better, 12-gauge) needle through the cricothyroid membrane into the trachea and connect it to an oxygen supply at 4 litres/min. (Use a 2 ml plastic syringe barrel to make a connector; attach the Luer tip to the cannula and the wide end to the oxygen tubing.) Delivering oxygen in this way will keep the patient alive for a few minutes, while you quickly consider whether the patency of the airway can be restored by changing the position of the patient, by allowing the patient to wake up, or by performing an emergency tracheostomy. (If you have given suxamethonium its effects should wear off within a few minutes, allowing the patient to breathe.)

If you can ventilate the lungs with a face mask, the patient's condition is much more stable. Give the patient at least 10 good breaths of oxygen, and at the same time look again at the position of the head and neck. The head should be extended and the neck slightly flexed (Fig. 2.1).

The commonest causes of failed intubation are (a) overextension of the neck, which pulls the larynx away from the mouth, and (b) putting the laryngoscope blade in too fast and too far (without identifying the uvula and epiglottis) and passing the laryngeal opening without seeing it.

Having repositioned the head, if necessary, and ensured oxygenation, you should make only one more attempt at intubation, following the procedures shown in Fig. 2.6. Put the laryngoscope blade in slowly (you may need to suck out secretions) and find the uvula and epiglottis. If you can identify the two arytenoid cartilages, which lie at the back of the larynx, pass the tube between and in front of them. If you cannot identify the arytenoid cartilages, ask your assistant to press gently on the thyroid cartilage and to retract the patient's upper lip to improve your view, and then insert the tube. It is helpful to use a gum-elastic bougie as a stylet over which the tube can be guided.

Check again whether the tube is in the trachea. If you are not sure, you must remove the tube.

Failed intubation drill

If you have not succeeded in intubating the patient, you must keep the airway clear by another means. If anaesthesia is necessary, adopt the *failed intubation drill* as follows.

- If the patient has a full stomach, your assistant must maintain cricoid pressure (see page 77) throughout the operation.
- Allow the patient to breathe, with an airway inserted if this is of help, and give an inhalational anaesthetic with a face mask. If profound relaxation is required, use 6–10% ether preceded by halothane for a few minutes, if available, to settle the patient. As soon as possible, turn the patient into the lateral position with 10–15 degrees of head-down tilt; it may even be possible to do the operation in this position.
- At the end of the procedure when the patient has recovered, try to determine the specific cause of the difficulty in intubation, so that you can avoid it in the future.

Care of the patient whose breathing is inadequate

Once you are sure that the airway is clear, check that the patient is breathing adequately. The signs of inadequate or absent breathing are:

- central cyanosis
- no breath heard or felt at the mouth or nose
- no activity of the respiratory muscles.

If these signs are present you must ventilate the lungs immediately by using one of the following techniques.

Ventilation with expired air without intubation

Your own expired air contains 16% oxygen, which is enough to maintain adequate oxygenation in the apnoeic patient. If you have no ventilating apparatus nearby, start with mouth-to-mouth ventilation (Fig. 2.7): check again that the airway is clear and extend the patient's head; pinch the nostrils, place your mouth over the patient's mouth, and blow into the lungs; watch the chest rise during inspiration; then lift your head and watch the chest wall fall with expiration. When you are ventilating a child's lungs in this way, it is easier to cover both the nose and the mouth with your mouth. Aim for a respiratory rate of 15 breaths per minute in an adult and about 30–40 in a child.

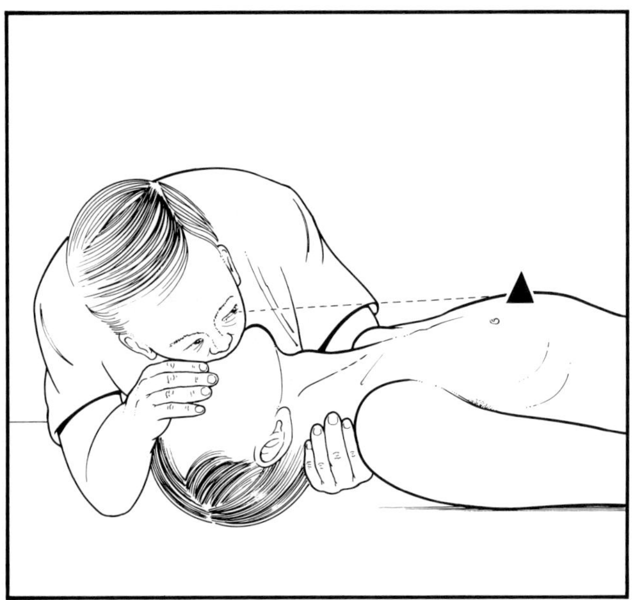

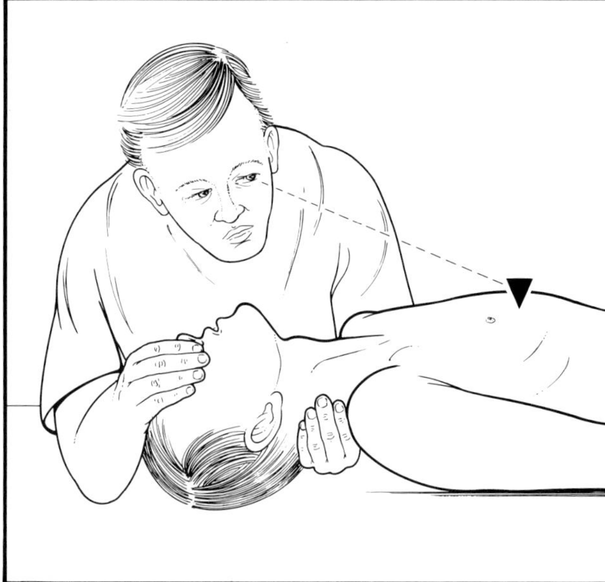

Fig. 2.7. Ventilation with expired air.

If possible, you should insert an oropharyngeal airway to help keep the airway clear (see page 13). If an anaesthetic face mask is available, it will make your task easier and more pleasant; use the mask as for an anaesthetic to cover the patient's mouth and nose, and support the jaw at the same time. To inflate the patient's lungs, blow through the hole in the mask. (Brook's double-ended airways are available for the same purpose, but are more difficult to use, and most anaesthetists prefer the face mask.)

Ventilation with an SIB without intubation

Air (or oxygen-enriched air) is drawn into an SIB through a non-return valve, and when the bellows or bag is compressed, the contents are driven into the patient's lungs via a breathing valve and face mask. Some examples of SIBs are shown in Fig. 2.8.

The breathing valve directs air from the SIB into the lungs during inspiration and allows the patient's expired air to pass out into the atmosphere during expiration. The valves shown in Fig. 2.9 are "universal", which means that they can be used for both controlled breathing (intermittent positive pressure ventilation, IPPV) and spontaneous breathing. They are therefore used for both resuscitation and anaesthesia. Check that you have the right sort of valve, if necessary by blowing and breathing through it yourself. The direction of air flow should be as shown in Fig. 2.9.

Connect the SIB via the breathing valve to the face mask. Ensure that the patient has a clear airway and inflate the lungs about 15 times per minute (30–40 times per minute for a child). Allow the patient to breathe out for about twice as long as it takes to inflate the lungs. To ventilate a child's lungs, use a smaller SIB if available or a smaller "squeeze" on an adult-size SIB, or use the mouth-to-mask/tube method. Oxygen enrichment is always desirable during resuscitation. The simplest and most economical way of providing it is by using a T-piece and reservoir tube at the inlet of the SIB (Fig. 2.10). An alternative can be improvised, if necessary, from any piece of wide-bore tubing with a piece of oxygen tubing running into it. A flow of 1–2 litres/min of oxygen into such a reservoir will increase the oxygen concentration in the inspired gas to 40–50%.

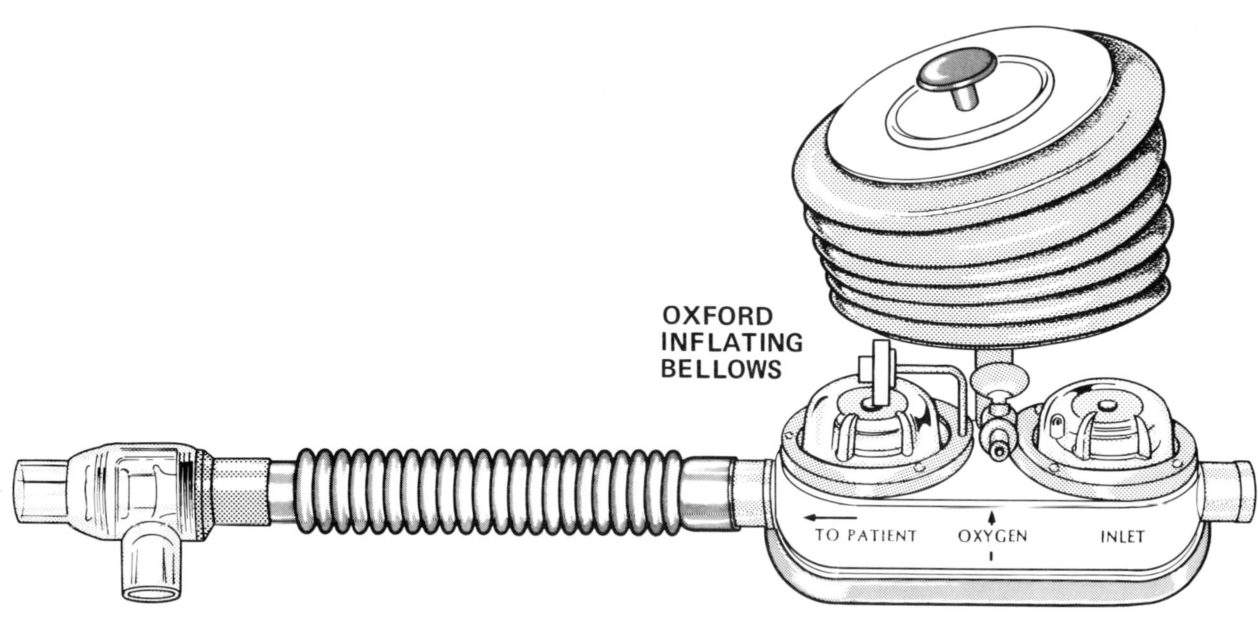

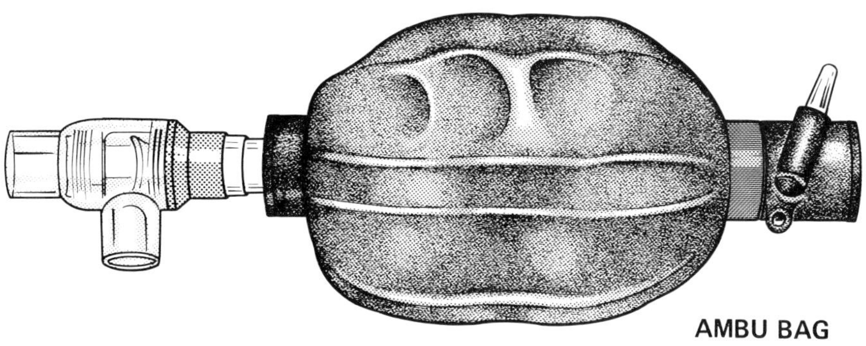

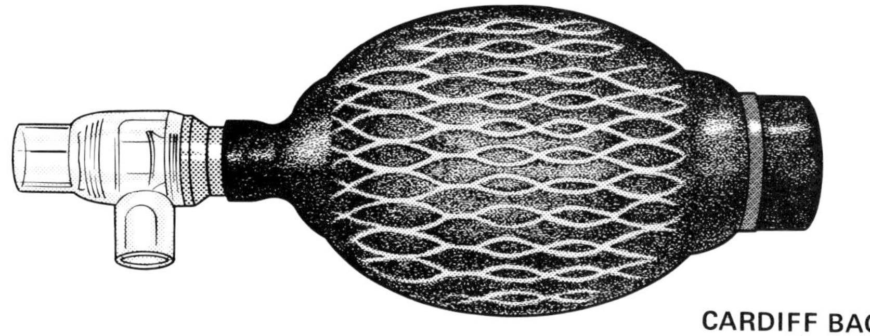

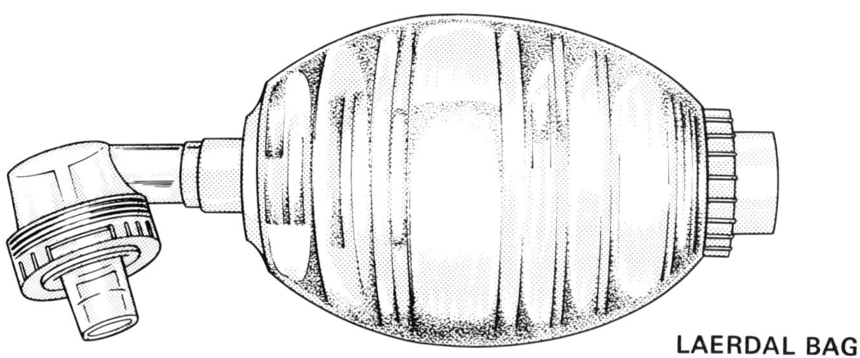

Fig. 2.8. Apparatus for ventilating the lungs (SIB).

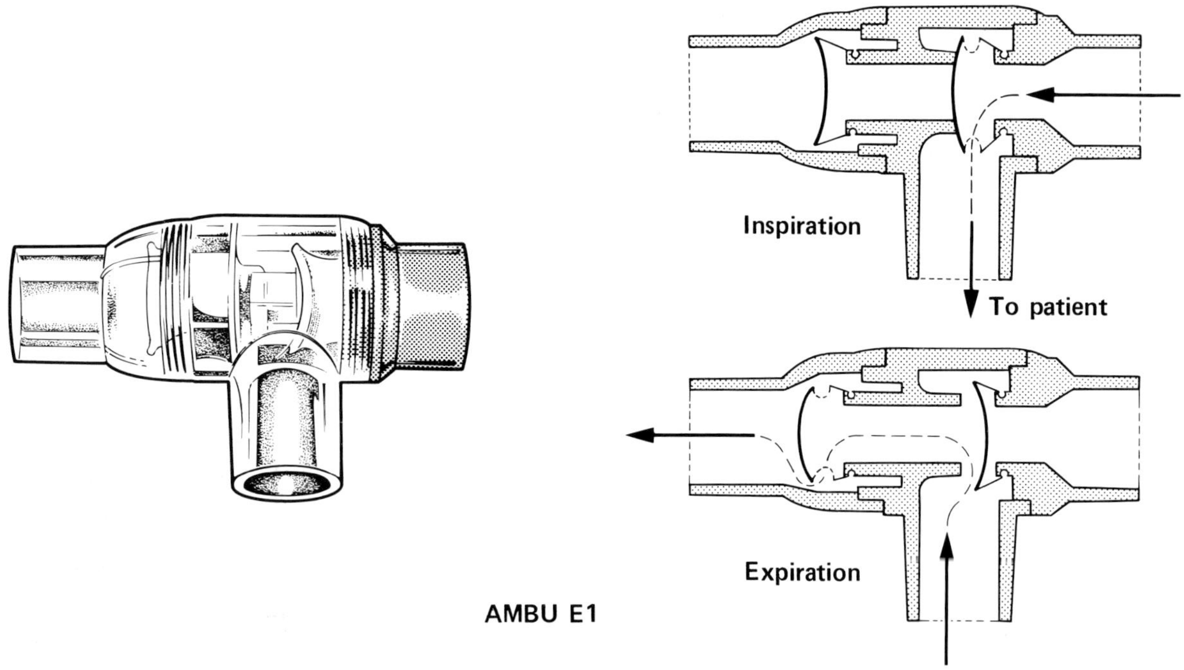

Inspiration

To patient

Expiration

AMBU E1

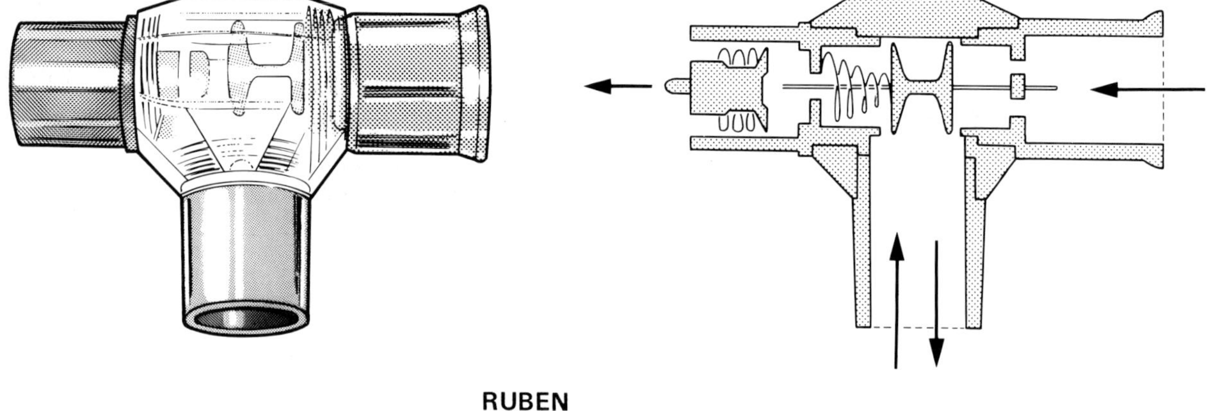

RUBEN

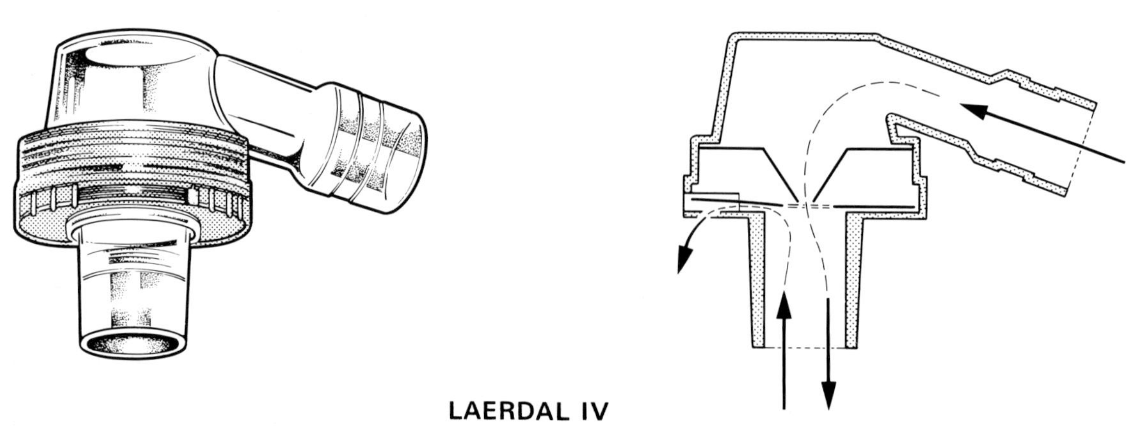

LAERDAL IV

Fig. 2.9. Universal breathing valves.

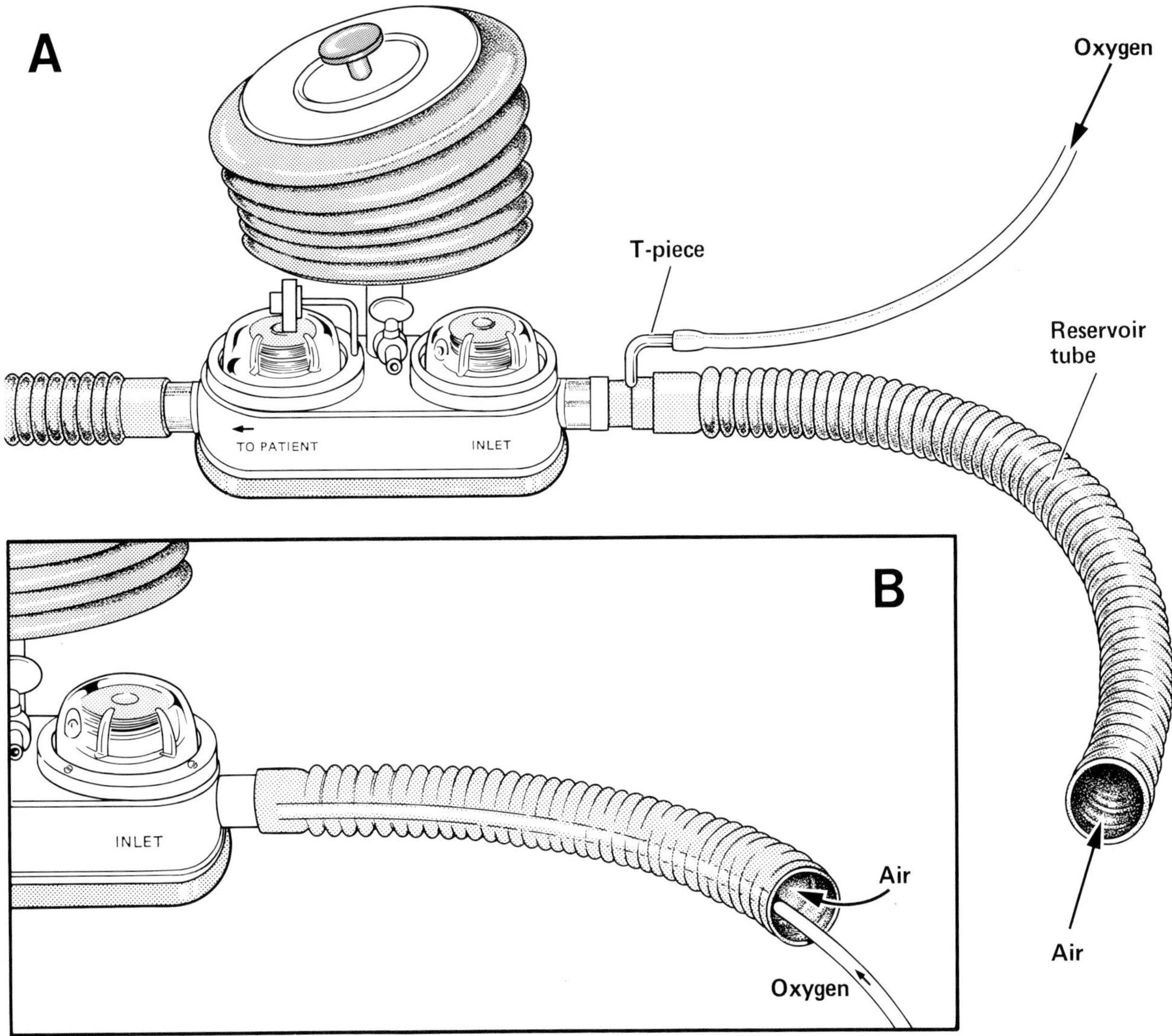

Fig. 2.10. **Oxygen enrichment of gas for ventilation with a self-inflating bellows. (A) A T-piece and reservoir tube; (B) an improvised alternative.**

Ventilation with an SIB with intubation

Before intubation you should always inflate the patient's lungs for a few breaths using either a mouth-to-mouth or a face-mask technique; oxygenation always has priority over intubation, since the latter may take several minutes and the patient may otherwise become hypoxic. Intubation is desirable if you are giving IPPV with an SIB, since it ensures a stable, clear airway and also provides invaluable protection against contamination of the lungs with vomit. Remember that, in deeply unconscious patients, no relaxant drugs are needed for laryngoscopy and intubation.

Management of the circulation

Immediate access to the circulation, i.e., a secure intravenous line, is needed in all critically ill and anaesthetized patients. In the critically ill adult, set up an infusion of an appropriate fluid into a large vein using the largest cannula or needle you have (14-gauge/2 mm is ideal). In some patients, two or more intravenous lines may be needed. If peripheral veins are invisible or inadequate, use large veins in the cubital fossa, the external or internal jugular veins, or even, for short-term use, the femoral vein (but beware of inserting the needle into the artery by mistake). If available, an extra assistant may do a surgical "cut-down" to provide access to the long saphenous vein, but this takes longer.

Control of bleeding

Bleeding from wounds can usually be controlled by firm pressure over a sterile dressing until the patient is ready for surgical exploration and haemostasis. However, some limb wounds, for example a severe crush injury, may need a temporary tourniquet.

Restoration of circulating volume

Elevating the legs will often improve venous return in the hypovolaemic patient. Doing this without lowering the trunk and head will avoid the impairment of breathing that is a feature of the head-down (Trendelenburg) position.

Further restoration of volume can be achieved by the intravenous infusion of fluids. The low blood pressure and cardiac output of hypovolaemia, whether caused by haemorrhage or by dehydration, can rapidly cause severe and irreversible damage to sensitive tissues, such as the kidney and brain, unless circulating volume is rapidly restored. The best fluid to give is one that resembles as closely as possible the fluid lost. It is reasonable to start resuscitation with a solution roughly equivalent to extracellular fluid, for example physiological (normal) saline or Ringer's lactate solution (Hartmann's solution). Metabolic acidosis often complicates severe circulatory failure; if it is severe, sodium bicarbonate may be given intravenously in a dose of 1 mmol/kg of body weight, except to patients with diabetic ketoacidosis in whom bicarbonate can precipitate fatal hypokalaemia.

For the management of unexpected cardiorespiratory arrest, see page 39.

Assessment of the effects of treatment

Failure of the circulation or breathing results in tissue hypoxia and cyanosis (unless the patient is also very anaemic, when cyanosis may not be detectable). While you are continuing with resuscitation of any unconscious patient, note whether the patient's colour and peripheral perfusion improve. If you are performing external cardiac massage (see page 40), a femoral pulse should be palpable if the massage is effective. If the patient's colour does not improve quickly, check that you have not forgotten part of the procedure or the assessment. If your resuscitation is effective, the patient will begin to regain consciousness and will start to move, breathe, or respond to stimulation. If the patient starts to breathe, continue to assist breathing until it is regular and adequate, i.e., occurs at a normal rate and depth, and the patient shows no cyanosis. You may then stop artificial ventilation, but continue to give oxygen. If the patient has been intubated, do not remove the endotracheal tube. It can be safely left in place until the patient is awake enough to remove it.

Monitor and record the pulse and blood pressure during resuscitation and adjust your treatment accordingly. If the heart rate is under 50 beats/min (100 in a baby) atropine may improve it and increase the cardiac output, and is unlikely to harm the patient. When possible, an electrocardiogram (ECG) should be obtained to provide specific diagnosis of abnormal cardiac rhythms, for which appropriate treatment can be given.

A urinary catheter should be inserted if the patient is severely hypovolaemic. The production of a urine volume of more than 0.5 ml/kg of body weight per hour is a good indicator that fluid replacement and cardiac output are adequate. Watch also for a rise in the jugular venous pressure, as this indicates that the venous circulation has been adequately filled. A patient who remains anuric (check that the catheter has not been blocked) despite normal blood pressure and jugular venous pressure has developed acute renal failure and must be referred immediately.

Stabilization of the patient

After initial resuscitation of the patient, further assessment and treatment will be needed while resuscitation continues. The treatment may include urgent surgical procedures such as insertion of chest drains, further control of bleeding, wound débridement, immobilization of fractures, and control of pain. Any of these procedures may result in further decompensation of the cardiovascular or respiratory systems, so continued monitoring of vital signs is important. If anaesthesia is necessary, it is vital to restore the patient's circulation to normal before induction. *Above all, the hypovolaemic patient should never be given a spinal anaesthetic, or fatal cardiovascular collapse may follow.*

Transportation of the critically ill patient

After initial resuscitation, the patient will need to be moved to an operating theatre or a ward, or possibly to another hospital for further treatment. Before any such move, the patient's condition must be reasonably stable. The active treatment and monitoring of a patient are more difficult during transportation than in the emergency room, so for any but the shortest journeys you should consider taking additional precautions. If the security of the airway is in any doubt, you should either intubate the patient or perform an elective tracheostomy. Think again about the need for a chest drain in the traumatized patient, and ensure good immobilization and pain relief for fractures. (Unstable fractures can cause renewed bleeding.) The safest way to give potent analgesics is by intravenous injection of small doses. Do not give analgesics or other depressant drugs to patients with impaired consciousness, or you will make any brain injury worse and possibly fatal. Evaluate the need for a regional anaesthetic block, for example a femoral nerve block for a fractured femur (see page 96).

You must also decide what equipment should accompany the patient. For any journey of more than a few minutes you will probably need all the resuscitation equipment mentioned so far (laryngoscope, endotracheal tube, SIB, intravenous infusion apparatus, etc.) together with supplies of any drugs that may be needed in transit. Most important is the choice of who should accompany the patient, although your choice may be limited. If possible go yourself, or send a nurse or trained assistant familiar with the techniques and apparatus of resuscitation and monitoring.

When to abandon resuscitation

Resuscitation is a very active form of treatment that aims to save the lives of severely ill or injured patients who are capable of subsequent recovery. It may be inappropriate to start this treatment at all in certain patients with progressive and incurable illnesses. It is also pointless to continue resuscitation of a patient for whom, despite your best efforts, there is no hope of recovery. The decision to stop resuscitation is a clinical one, based on examination of the patient. The following points may be useful as a guide.

1. A patient who has fixed, dilated pupils *and* stops breathing (but whose airway is not obstructed) after a head injury is unlikely to survive.
2. The following signs, if present after 30 min of intensive resuscitation, indicate a poor prognosis:
   - fixed and dilated pupils
   - impalpable femoral and carotid pulses
   - absence of respiration.

If these signs are all present there is no hope of recovery, and resuscitation should be abandoned.

The severely injured patient

When a severely injured patient is admitted to the hospital, it may sometimes be difficult to know where to start. The initial priorities of course are management of the airway, breathing, and circulation. The aim of this section is to give you more specific guidance about the further management of particular injuries.

Injuries of the head and neck

The commonest cause of death after head injury is an obstructed airway, so make sure that your patient's airway is clear. You must protect the airway of an unconscious patient by turning him or her into the semiprone position or by inserting a cuffed endotracheal tube. If you suspect an injury of the cervical spine, try to maintain the head and neck in a neutral or slightly extended position, and make sure that enough assistants are present to turn the patient without twisting the neck. Flexion is the manoeuvre most likely to damage the spinal cord after a cervical fracture. If endotracheal intubation is necessary in such a patient, for example to allow the surgeon to perform a laparotomy for suspected bleeding, a skilled assistant — the surgeon is best — should hold the head and neck firmly in a safe position while you perform the laryngoscopy and intubation. Do not hesitate to intubate if necessary, especially for anaesthesia. You are much more likely to damage the patient's neck if you try to give an anaesthetic with a face mask, and will also expose the patient to the dangers of regurgitated stomach contents. Avoid nasotracheal intubation, as there may be a basal skull fracture through which you could introduce infection by inserting the tube.

If spinal injuries are suspected and it is necessary to turn the patient, you will need at least four people to "log-roll" him or her, avoiding any twisting of the spine from head to coccyx. A patient who needs to be transported should be put on a firm surface and stabilized in position with pillows or sandbags.

Remember that the patient with a spinal cord injury may develop "spinal shock" because of loss of vasoconstrictor tone and that the blood pressure may be extremely sensitive to changes in position. Give generous fluid therapy if this is so, and insert a urinary catheter.

Bleeding from the scalp can be very severe, so make sure that firm pressure is applied. Radiographs of the skull are unlikely to be helpful in the immediate management of most patients with head injuries. A patient who is totally unresponsive to stimulation and who has fixed and dilated pupils probably has a very severe brain injury, and if such a patient stops breathing (after you have ensured a clear airway by intubation) then further resuscitation is pointless. In less severely injured patients a clear airway is vital, since obstructed breathing, hypoxia, and hypercapnia all increase intracranial pressure and thus cause further cerebral damage. Any patient with head injuries and impaired consciousness who needs to be transported must first undergo intubation or tracheostomy.

Chest injuries

Any patient who has fractured ribs can develop a pneumothorax or haemopneumothorax, which requires the emergency insertion of a chest drain. Look for the signs of diminished chest movement and air entry, and a deviated trachea. The physical signs may be difficult to interpret, so you should always obtain a radiograph of the chest as soon as possible. If this confirms pneumothorax or haemopneumothorax, insert a chest drain, connected to an underwater seal, and obtain a second radiograph. Penetrating chest wounds must rapidly be made airtight by a temporary dressing. Any patient with a flail segment — an area of the chest wall that is unstable and moves inward during inspiration — is in severe danger. Give oxygen, and if respiratory distress persists, proceed to endotracheal intubation and IPPV before transferring the patient to a larger hospital. (This type of injury may require IPPV for up to 2 weeks.) A patient with a small flail segment who is not in respiratory distress will often do well if given adequate analgesia to alleviate rib pain, which inhibits deep breathing and coughing. For analgesia, consider regular intercostal blocks (see page 95) with bupivacaine or, for the regular physiotherapy the patient will need, inhalational analgesia with 0.5% trichloroethylene or 50% nitrous oxide in oxygen.

Abdominal injuries

There may be intra-abdominal bleeding or rupture of a viscus, without any obvious evidence of external abdominal injury. Intra-abdominal bleeding may be confirmed by peritoneal lavage with saline, but a negative result does not necessarily exclude it, especially if bleeding is retroperitoneal. Always suspect intra-abdominal bleeding in cases of multiple trauma, especially if the visible injuries fail to account for the patient's pulse and blood pressure.

Major fractures

Remember that fractures, whether closed or compound, can be a major source of blood loss: 2–3 litres from a severe pelvic fracture and 1–2 litres from a fractured femur. Immobilize fractures as soon as possible, for example using a Thomas' splint for a fractured femur, and give appropriate fluid replacement and analgesia. Administering small doses of opiates intravenously will often be the safest and most effective analgesic technique. For a fractured femur, a femoral nerve block is simple and safe (see page 96).

Burn injuries

Burned patients may have hidden injuries from the inhalation of hot or toxic gases. Those with burns of the upper respiratory tract (which may quickly lead to fatal laryngeal oedema) may also have burns of the face and singed nasal hair. Steroids are recommended to control oedema, but if they are not rapidly effective, early endotracheal intubation or tracheostomy will be required. Oxygen therapy should be given to any patient suspected of having burns of the respiratory tract. Inhalation of smoke or toxic fumes may cause a chemical pneumonitis with severe hypoxia, requiring long-term IPPV. Patients with burns of the respiratory tract should be referred as soon as their condition can be stabilized, which should usually be within 24 hours of injury. Patients with severe pain should be given small intravenous doses of morphine or pethidine until their pain is relieved.

For external burns make an estimate of the percentage area burned. For an adult use the "rule of nines". Each of the following areas can be taken as 9% of the total body area: front of thorax, back of thorax, front of abdomen, back of abdomen, each arm, front of each leg, back of each leg, head plus neck. The area of the perineum is about 1% of the total. For children the area of the head is proportionately much greater, for example 15% for a 5-year-old and 20% for a 1-year-old. Another useful measure is the front of the patient's hand, which usually represents about 1% of the surface area.

Set up an intravenous infusion into a large vein and give fluid replacement as suggested below. Severely burned patients lose blood and protein through the burned surface and must be given colloids and blood as necessary, in addition to the extra saline and water needed to replace excess water losses due to evaporation from burned areas and a very high metabolic rate. Keep the patient in as warm an environment as possible to minimize the metabolic disturbance. Measure hourly urinary output as an index of the adequacy of your fluid therapy and try to maintain a urine flow of at least 0.5 ml/kg of body weight per hour. It is helpful to measure central venous pressure, which should be maintained at 10–20 cmH_2O (0.98–1.96 kPa) above the right atrium. The erythrocyte volume fraction should be kept if possible in the range 0.30–0.35 (haematocrit 30–35%).

Suggested fluid regimen

When you have assessed the area of the burn, use your estimate to determine the "unit of fluid replacement" from the formula:

1 unit of replacement (ml) = total area of burns × body weight in kg × 0.5

For example, for a 30% burn in a 60 kg adult the unit of replacement would be 30 × 60 × 0.5 = 900 ml. Give the replacement fluid as colloid (dextran, polygeline, hydroxyethyl starch, plasma, or blood) according to the following schedule:

1 unit every 4 hours for the first 12 hours
1 unit every 6 hours for the next 12 hours
1 unit during the next 12 hours
(total 6 units of replacement in 36 hours)

In addition, give the daily water requirement of the patient orally, or intravenously as a 5% (50 g/litre) glucose solution (at least 35 ml/kg of body weight per day for adults and 150 ml/kg of body weight per day for children weighing less than 10 kg).

If the sum of the area burned (as a percentage) and the patient's age exceeds 100, the patient is unlikely to survive, but make sure that he or she is comfortable by giving generous doses of opiate analgesics. Patients who survive a severe burn will have a very catabolic metabolism, but will also be anorexic, and will starve to death unless you make a special effort to feed them. This will usually mean the need for nasogastric feeding with a high protein and high calorie diet — up to 25.1 MJ/day (6000 $kcal_{th}$/day). Repeated anaesthetics may be needed later for painful dressings and skin grafts. Ketamine is very valuable in this situation, as is inhalational analgesia with trichloroethylene. Never give suxamethonium to a patient after a severe burn, as it may cause the release of large quantities of potassium ions into the circulation, resulting in cardiac arrest.

3
Care of unconscious and anaesthetized patients

The previous chapter outlined the steps to be taken for the immediate care of critically ill or unconscious patients. This chapter now focuses on the continuing care of unconscious and anaesthetized patients.

A person who is unconscious, whether because of injury or illness or because of the influence of general anaesthetic drugs, lacks many vital and protective reflexes and depends on other people for protection and maintenance of vital functions. It is a doctor's duty to ensure that the patient is protected during this critical period. One person must never act as both anaesthetist and surgeon at the same time; a trained person must always be available specifically to look after the airway, monitor the patient, and care for all vital functions.

General management

Position

Patients, whether awake or asleep, must be handled gently at all times. Anaesthesia should always be induced with the patient on a table or trolley that can rapidly be tilted into a steep, head-down position to deal with any sudden onset of hypotension or, should the patient vomit, to allow the vomit to drain out of the mouth instead of into the lungs. General anaesthesia is usually induced with the patient in the supine position, but if you are planning to anaesthetize the patient in the lateral position without an endotracheal tube, anaesthesia can be induced with the patient already in that position.

Once anaesthetized, the patient should not be put into abnormal positions that could cause damage to joints or muscles. If the lithotomy position is to be used, two assistants should lift both legs at the same time and place them in the stirrups, to avoid damage to the sacro-iliac joint.

Eyes

The eyes should be fully closed during general anaesthesia or the cornea may become dry and ulcerated. If the lids do not close "naturally", a small piece of tape should be used to hold them. They should always be taped in this way if the head is to be draped, and additional protective padding is advisable. If the patient is to be placed in the prone position, special care is also needed to prevent pressure on the eyes, which could permanently damage vision.

Teeth

The teeth are at risk from artificial airways and laryngoscopy, especially if they are loose, decayed, or irregularly spaced. Damage from oral airways most often occurs during recovery from anaesthesia, when an increase in muscle tone causes the patient to bite. Laryngoscopy may damage teeth, particularly the upper front incisors, if they are used as a fulcrum on which to lever the laryngoscope. It is safer to remove a loose tooth deliberately, because if dislodged by accident it may be inhaled and result in a lung abscess.

Peripheral nerves

Certain peripheral nerves (for example the ulnar nerve at the elbow) may be damaged by prolonged pressure, and others (for example the brachial plexus) by traction. Careful attention to the patient's position and the use of soft padding over bony prominences can avoid these problems. Tourniquets, if used, must be carefully applied with padding and must never be left inflated for more than 90 min, or ischaemic nerve damage can result.

Breathing

Unrestricted breathing is essential for the unconscious patient. Make sure that the surgeon's assistant is not leaning on the chest wall or upper abdomen. Steep, head-down positions restrict movement of the diaphragm, especially in obese patients, and controlled ventilation may therefore be necessary. If a patient is placed in the prone position, insert pillows under the upper chest and pelvis to allow free movement of the abdominal wall during respiration.

Thermal injury

Protect the anaesthetized patient from being burned accidentally. Beware of inflammable skin-cleaning solutions that can be ignited by surgical diathermy. To prevent diathermy burns, apply the neutral diathermy electrode firmly and evenly to a large area of skin over the back, buttock, or thigh. If other electrical apparatus is in use, beware of the risk of electrocuting or electrically burning the patient.

Heat loss

Keep unconscious patients as warm as possible by covering them and keeping them out of draughts. Most general and regional anaesthetics cause skin vasodilatation, which increases heat loss from the body. Although the skin feels warm, the patient's core temperature may be falling rapidly. Hypothermia during anaesthesia has two harmful effects: it increases and prolongs the effects of certain drugs (for example muscle relaxants) and, by causing the patient to shiver during the recovery period, it increases oxygen demand, which can lead to hypoxia.

Respiratory function in the anaesthetized patient

The principles of keeping a clear airway (described on page 12) apply as much to the anaesthetized patient as to any unconscious or severely injured patient. Many short or minor surgical procedures, for example incision and drainage, can be carried out with the patient in the lateral or semiprone position, which gives added protection to the airway. If general anaesthesia is needed for intermediate or major procedures, endotracheal anaesthesia should normally be used.

General anaesthesia often impairs the function of the lungs, particularly if the patient is permitted to breathe spontaneously after having been given respiratory depressant drugs, such as morphine or halothane. Very close monitoring of the respiratory system is therefore necessary, though no special or complicated equipment is required. Watch the patient constantly, noting in particular any change in colour or chest movement.

Provided that the patient is not severely anaemic, a healthy pink colour of mucous membranes, fingers, and toes indicates adequate oxygenation. Always make sure that a finger or toe protrudes from under the drapes so that you can observe its colour. Also look at the colour of blood in the surgical wound.

The chest should rise freely with inspiration and fall during expiration. Because the diaphragm descends during inspiration, the epigastric region also rises. If there is an obstruction of the airway, descent of the diaphragm during inspiration causes indrawing of the lower ribs and the tissues at the root of the neck, which is known as "paradoxical respiration".

If respiration is markedly depressed, there may be signs of carbon dioxide retention. Carbon dioxide itself is a depressant, but it causes the release of catecholamines, which produce tachycardia, hypertension, and sweating. They may also cause cardiac dysrhythmias, which can be particularly dangerous if the patient is also hypoxic.

The movement of air as the patient breathes can be monitored by watching the SIB, the breathing valve, or a wisp of thread attached at an appropriate point on the anaesthetic vaporizer (Fig. 3.1). Breathing can also be monitored continuously with a precordial or oesophageal stethoscope. The latter can be easily made by tying a finger from a rubber glove over the end of a stomach tube, passing the tube approximately half way down the oesophagus, and connecting the top end to a normal stethoscope in place of the chest piece (Fig. 3.2). A stethoscope allows the anaesthetist to monitor breath sounds and the respiratory and heart rates; it is simple and reliable and is strongly recommended for routine use. Many anaesthetists find that a monaural earpiece is more comfortable for prolonged monitoring.

During controlled ventilation, as you squeeze the bellows or bag, be alert for changes in resistance that may indicate obstruction or kinking of the tube, accidental disconnection from the patient, the onset of bronchospasm or coughing, or the development of a pneumothorax.

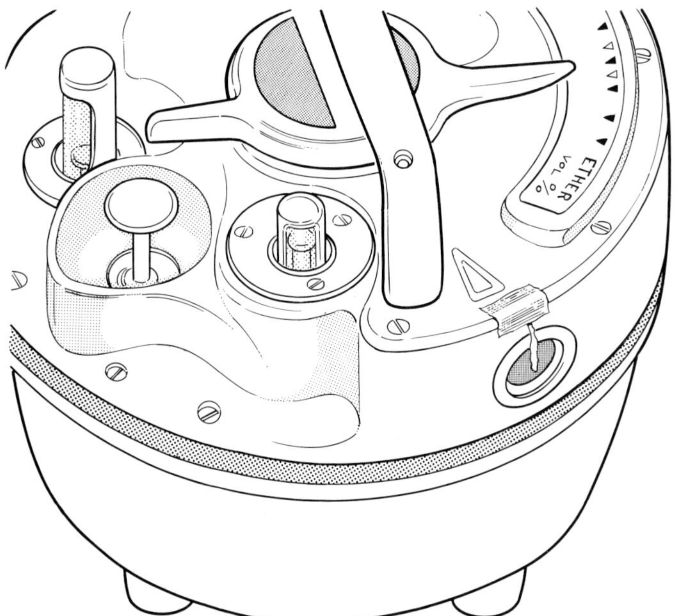

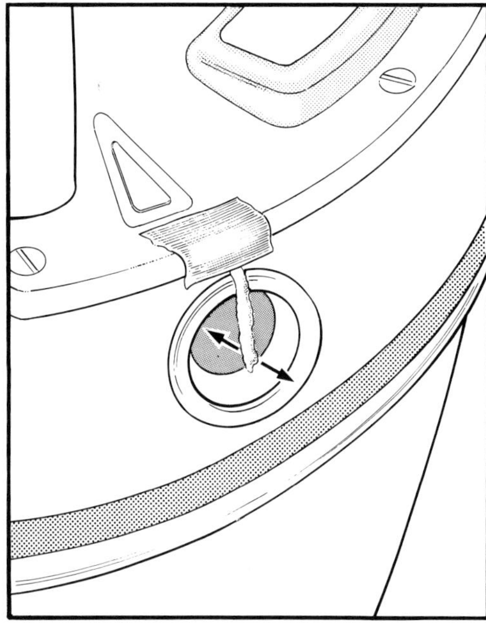

Fig. 3.1. A wisp of thread used as a simple monitor of respiration on a vaporizer.

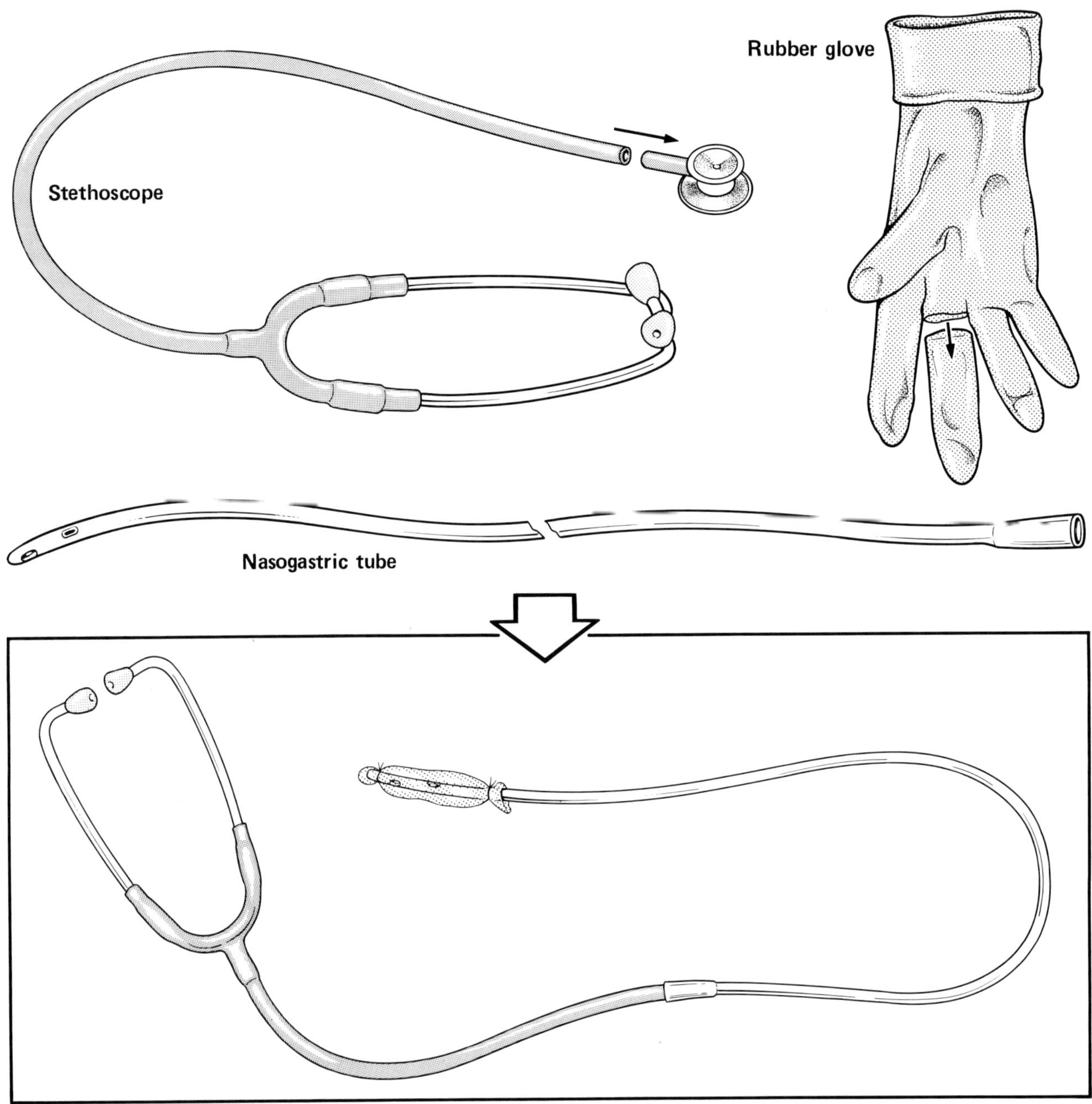

Fig. 3.2. Making an oesophageal stethoscope.

Mechanisms of respiratory obstruction

Obstruction of the upper airways during unconsciousness usually occurs because of loss of muscle tone and reflexes. Obstruction is more likely if the patient has a small lower jaw, a restricted mouth opening, a large tongue, an abnormality in the neck such as a large thyroid swelling, or an abnormal rigidity of the cervical spine. These abnormalities often lead to the tongue falling or being pressed back on to the posterior pharyngeal wall and blocking the passage of air. If this happens suddenly, for example after a bolus of drug has been injected intravenously to induce anaesthesia, and you can neither correct the problem nor ventilate the lungs with a face mask, the patient may die. This sort of sudden obstruction does not occur with inhalational induction of anaesthesia, which is more gradual than the intravenous method. Inhalational induction (see page 54) is therefore the only safe technique to use in a patient whose airway is difficult to manage.

If the patient is not intubated, the airway may also become obstructed as a result of laryngeal spasm, which can produce a "crowing" sound (stridor), especially on inspiration. There is a reflex increase in the force of contraction of the inspiratory muscles, resulting in indrawing of the tissues at the root of the neck and paradoxical movement of the ribs, i.e., inwards during inspiration. In patients with severe laryngeal spasm these signs are accentuated, but there is no sound since no air is moving through the larynx. Laryngeal spasm is usually a reflex response to stimulation during light anaesthesia. Either local stimulation (for example laryngoscopy with the patient too lightly anaesthetized) or painful surgical stimulation (for example forcible dilatation of the anal sphincter or cervix) may be responsible. If your patient develops laryngeal spasm, first remove any precipitating stimulus. After a few breaths, the spasm will usually become less marked; you can then deepen anaesthesia so that it will not recur when stimulation starts again. For severe spasm, give suxamethonium intravenously and insert an endotracheal tube. Probably the commonest cause of laryngeal spasm associated with anaesthesia is the removal of the endotracheal tube with the patient too lightly anaesthetized. To prevent the development of spasm at the end of anaesthesia, you should remove the endotracheal tube with the patient either deeply anaesthetized or fully awake.

Even after insertion of an endotracheal tube, obstruction may occur as a result of:

- a foreign body or dried mucus in the tube
- thick secretions in the patient's trachea
- kinking of the tube in the mouth or pharynx
- compression of the tube by a surgical gag
- pressure of the tube bevel against the tracheal wall
- herniation of the cuff over the end of the tube
- intubation of a bronchus (which is not really obstruction, but nevertheless causes high inflation pressure and cyanosis).

If after intubation your patient's airway appears to be obstructed, you must rapidly check for these possibilities and make appropriate corrections. In particular, check the patency of the tube by passing a suction catheter through it, check the position of the tube with a laryngoscope, and deflate the cuff in case it has herniated over the end of the tube.

If, after you have checked all these points, the patient's airway remains obstructed, you must remove the tube and begin again.

You can prevent certain types of obstruction by taking precautions when inserting the endotracheal tube. For example, if you use a stylet in the tube during intubation, you will insure against the presence of foreign bodies. It may also be helpful to cut a hole in the end of the endotracheal tube to facilitate air flow should the tube be badly positioned (Fig. 3.3 & 3.4).

Why is airway obstruction so dangerous?

Airway obstruction, if severe, always results in hypoxia, which damages all tissues, but is especially harmful to the heart, brain, and kidney. Minor degrees of hypoxia may be masked if the patient is receiving extra oxygen, but this does not prevent the accumulation of carbon dioxide in the tissues, with associated respiratory acidosis, hypertension, tachycardia, and cardiac dysrhythmias. In addition, the patient who is straining to overcome airway obstruction may generate a large pressure gradient between the thorax and abdomen, resulting in regurgitation of gastric contents into the oesophagus and lungs, with disastrous results.

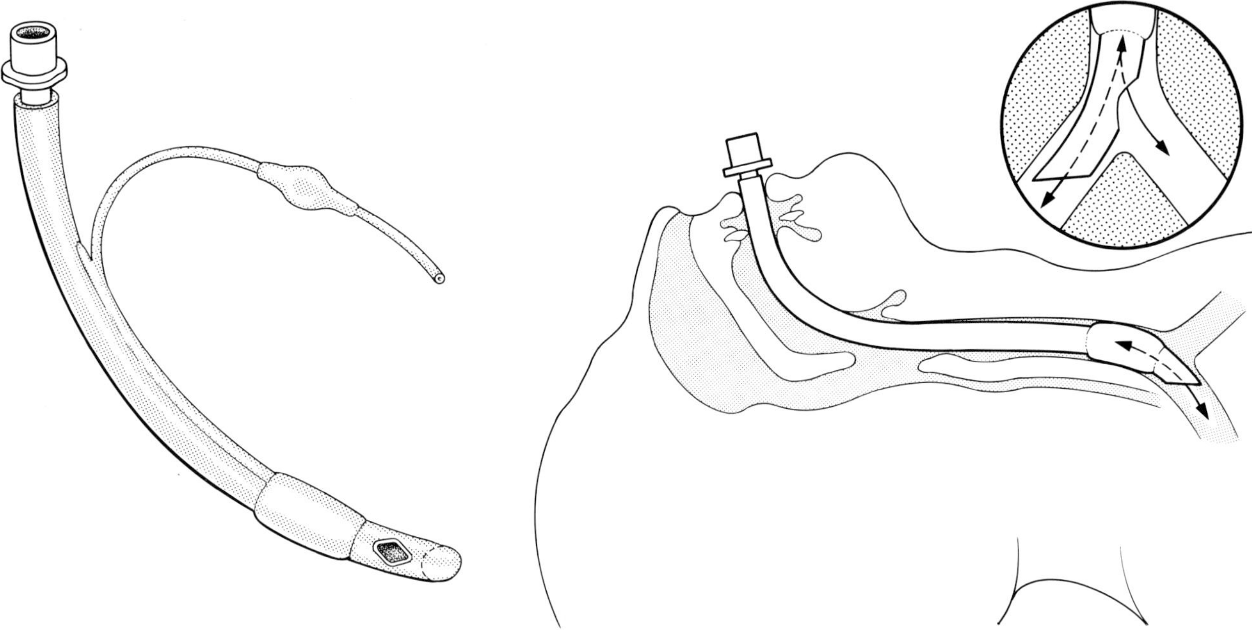

Fig. 3.3. Accidental intubation of a bronchus with a Magill's tube. The danger is less if a hole is cut in the side of the tube below the cuff.

Respiratory insufficiency

All drugs that depress the central nervous system (for example sedatives, analgesics, and inhalational and intravenous anaesthetics) are liable to produce some respiratory depression in the spontaneously breathing patient. The depressed respiratory centre fails to stimulate respiration in spite of an adequate stimulus (usually a rising level of arterial carbon dioxide), and the result is a variable degree of hypoxia, hypercapnia, and respiratory acidosis.

Certain factors make patients particularly susceptible to respiratory insufficiency. For example, severe brain injuries, such as those caused by trauma or by the hypoxia of a cardiac arrest, depress respiration and may even stop it. Patients with severe chronic obstruction of the airway, such as chronic bronchitis, also have abnormal respiratory responses and may be extremely sensitive to depressant drugs. In addition, patients who have received muscle relaxants are prone to respiratory insufficiency in the postoperative period if the effects of the relaxant have not been fully reversed at the end of anaesthesia. Certain drugs, if given in large doses during an operation (for example streptomycin at more than 20 mg/kg of body weight), potentiate the actions of muscle relaxants and may therefore accentuate respiratory depression.

In all cases of severe respiratory insufficiency, first give immediate artificial ventilation using a face mask or endotracheal tube to restore normal gas exchange. Drug-induced respiratory depression will eventually wear off if IPPV is continued for long enough. For patients suffering from opiate overdosage, use the specific antagonist naloxone, or nalorphine if available. Either of these drugs will reverse opiate-induced respiratory depression, though the effect may wear off before that of the depressant drug, so they must be used with care. Paralysis from muscle relaxants that persists after a normal dose of neostigmine may improve after a second dose of 0.04 mg/kg of body weight (see page 85). If respiration is still inadequate, continue IPPV until the paralysis wears off and do not give further doses of neostigmine. Persistent or recurrent paralysis is a particular problem in patients who become hypothermic during anaesthesia, since as they begin to warm up during the recovery period, the relaxant remaining in the body becomes more active, and produces so-called "re-curarization". Failure to breathe even after neostigmine has been given to reverse relaxant effects may also result from acidosis, hypokalaemia, and several fairly rare neurological conditions.

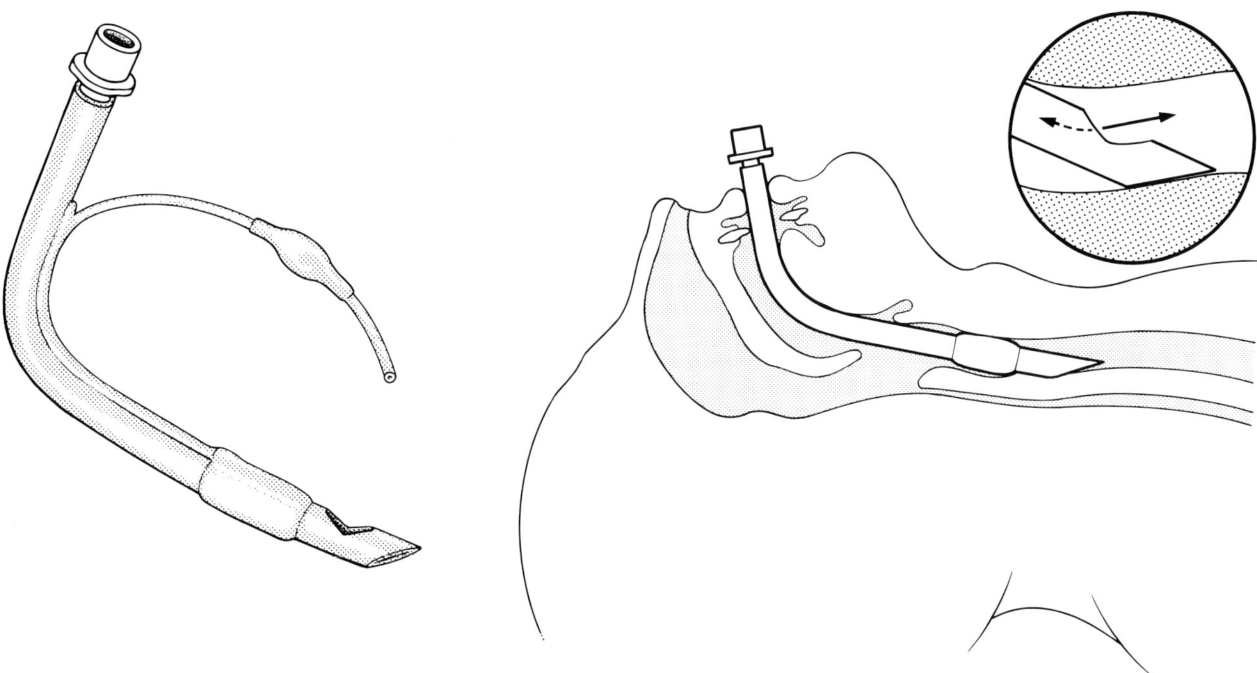

Fig. 3.4. Obstruction of the bevel of an Oxford tube can be prevented by cutting a hole in the lower part of the tube.

The cardiovascular system

It is vital at all stages of anaesthesia or unconsciousness to be aware of the condition of the patient's cardiovascular system. Blood flow through the tissues is of greatest importance, but in practice this can be estimated only indirectly from the patient's heart rate, blood pressure, peripheral colour and temperature, venous filling, and electrocardiogram. Observations and measurements should be made throughout anaesthesia and recorded on a chart similar to the one shown in the Annex 3. An accurate record of fluid and blood loss and fluid intake should also be kept. If you detect abnormalities you must inform the surgeon, who may need to take corrective action .

Heart rate

The heart rate can be simply counted by placing a finger over a suitable artery (during anaesthesia it is often easier to use the facial, superficial temporal, or carotid artery than the radial artery) or by listening with a precordial or oesophageal stethoscope. You should record the heart rate every 10 min if the patient's condition is stable, and more often if it is unstable. Tachycardia is usually an indication of increasing activity of the sympathetic nervous system and may indicate hypovolaemia due to excessive fluid or blood loss. Alternatively, it may mean that the patient is becoming too lightly anaesthetized and requires a further dose of anaesthetic drug; in this case the tachycardia is often accompanied by an increase in blood pressure. Bradycardia is usually a reflex response mediated through the vagus nerve; it may occur as a response to visceral stimulation such as traction on the mesentery or dilatation of the cervix. In small children and neonates, bradycardia may indicate hypoxia, which demands immediate correction (see page 115).

The heart rate is best monitored continuously. The simplest way to do this is with a stethoscope, but in some hospitals a simple, battery-operated pulse monitor may be available. The latter detects pulsatile blood flow in a finger or ear lobe and may display a flashing light with each pulsation, as well as a reading of the heart rate on a dial or display.

Blood pressure

Blood pressure is most conveniently measured using a cuff, which should be of the right size for the patient. (The width should be between a third and half the distance from elbow to shoulder.) Systolic pressure can be detected by palpation of the brachial or radial artery or by auscultation. In anaesthetic practice, the systolic pressure has greater significance than the diastolic pressure, which is frequently not recorded, particularly if access to the arm is difficult. No "normal" blood pressure can be specified for the anaesthetized patient; in general the systolic pressure should be stable in the range 90–140 mmHg (12.0–18.7 kPa). Measuring the blood pressure of small children may be difficult unless an infant-size cuff is available; a simple technique is to squeeze the forearm firmly, inflate the cuff above systolic pressure, and then note the pressure during deflation at which the forearm flushes with blood. Systolic arterial blood pressure is normally lower in children (45–75 mmHg or 6.0–10.0 kPa in neonates).

Peripheral blood flow

Peripheral blood flow cannot be measured directly, but can be roughly estimated by observing the colour and temperature of the hands and feet. A patient with warm, pink extremities and a normal blood pressure usually has a good cardiac output. You should be aware however that certain anaesthetic drugs, for example halothane, are skin vasodilators, while others, for example ether and ketamine, are not. Remember also that carbon dioxide retention can produce bounding pulses and warm extremities.

A urinary catheter is simple and very useful for assessing cardiac output. Unless the patient is severely dehydrated, as shown by a high relative density (specific gravity) of the urine, the production of urine at a rate of at least 0.5 ml/hour per kilogram of body weight indicates an adequate cardiac output, and it is generally safe to give fluids intravenously until this level of urine production is achieved.

Venous pressure and filling

In a small hospital, measuring the central venous pressure may be difficult, but information can still be obtained by inspecting the patient's neck veins. Position the patient in bed with his or her trunk reclining at an angle of about 45 degrees to the horizontal. Inspect the neck for evidence of venous pulsation. If too large a volume of fluid has been transfused, the patient's neck veins will be filled to a height of more than 15 cm above the sternal angle. In extreme cases, pulsation will not be seen, as the veins will be distended to the top of the neck. In a patient who is not hypovolaemic, the neck veins will be empty in the 45-degree position, but will become filled as the patient is lowered to the supine position. In the severely hypovolaemic patient, the veins will remain empty, even when the patient is supine, and will fill only when the patient is in a head-down position.

The electrocardiogram

Continuous monitoring of the electrical activity of the heart during anaesthesia is not possible unless an electrocardiograph with screen display is available. A paper-writing electrocardiograph may still be of value in the operating theatre to help diagnose dysrhythmias, whose presence is first indicated by abnormalities of the pulse or changes in blood pressure. For patients with evidence of cardiac disease, a preoperative electrocardiogram should of course be recorded.

Intravenous access

Before giving a patient any kind of anaesthetic, whether general or regional, you must secure intravenous access with either a plastic intravenous cannula or an indwelling needle. In adults a large forearm vein is ideal for this. Avoid veins where they cross the wrist or elbow joints. In adults the external or internal jugular veins are useful, especially for resuscitation purposes, but use the internal jugular vein only if you have had thorough practical instruction from an experienced teacher. In small children scalp veins are often available. The femoral vein can be used in any patient if you find it difficult to gain access to another vein for resuscitation purposes, but because of greater risks of infection and thrombosis, you should always re-site your infusion within a few hours. (See also page 25 for intravenous access for emergency procedures.)

Management of unexpected cardiorespiratory arrest

If any patient suddenly develops a cardiorespiratory arrest, treatment is extremely urgent; irreversible brain damage will occur if the oxygen supply to the brain is cut off for more than 3 min. It is possible to maintain the circulation and ventilation of the lungs by active resuscitation while the underlying cause of the arrest is treated, and many patients recover well after such treatment. If you are inexperienced, the main problem may well be in deciding whether to start resuscitation. Remember that a patient who has a cardiac arrest cannot survive unless treated, so do not delay. When faced with a collapsed patient, first check the *airway*, *breathing*, and *circulation* (this takes about 15 s). If you diagnose a cardiac arrest:

1. Start resuscitation. Don't leave the patient. Shout "Help — cardiac arrest" until help arrives.
2. Clear the airway and inflate the lungs with whatever means is available: your own expired air; a bag or bellows; or oxygen.

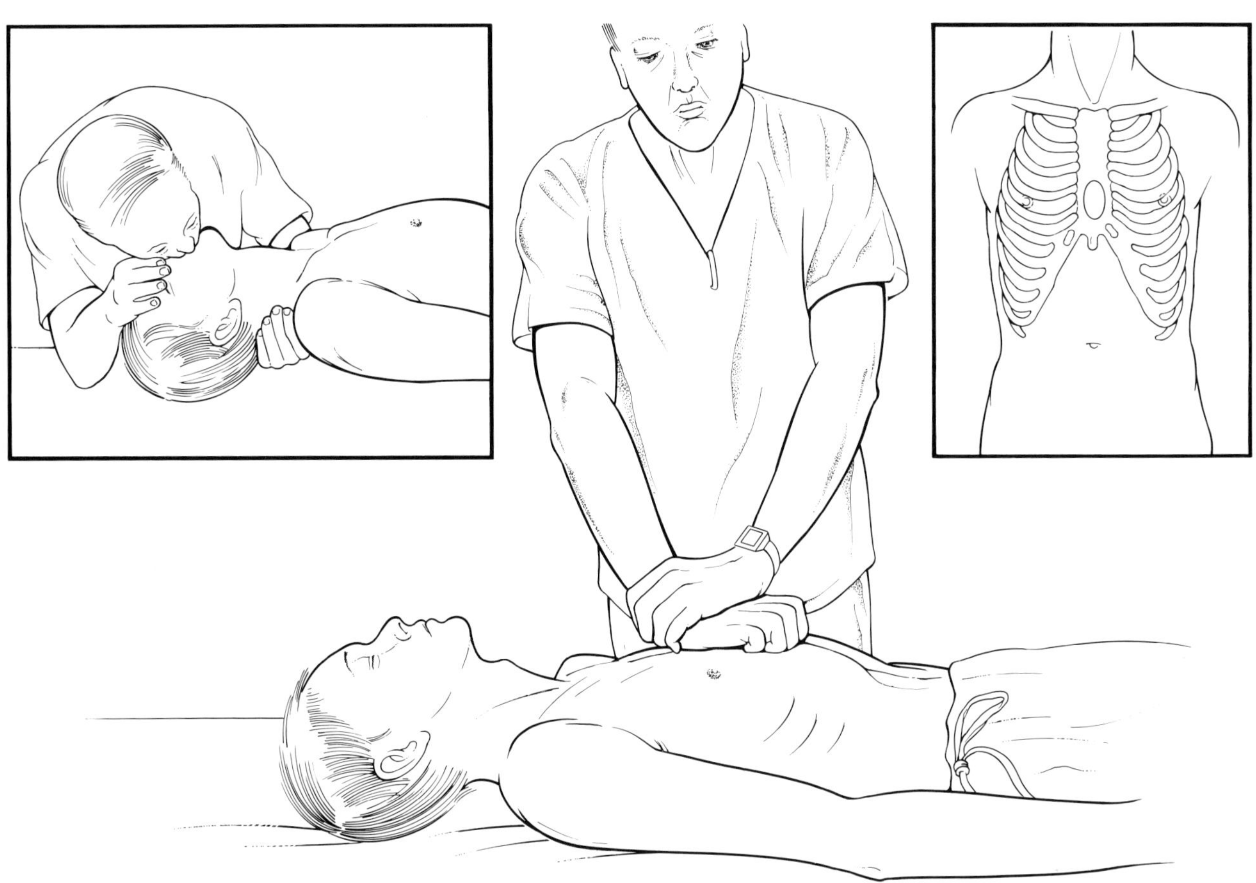

Fig. 3.5. Expired-air resuscitation and external cardiac massage. The oval marked on the sternum in the drawing on the right shows where pressure should be applied.

3. If there is no major pulse, start external cardiac massage. With one hand on top of the other, press sharply down on the lower third of the sternum in the midline (Fig. 3.5); this compresses and empties the heart between the sternum and vertebral column. Do not massage the left chest, as this does not compress the heart effectively and is more likely to break the ribs. A massage rate of 60 per minute for adults and up to 120 per minute for small children is appropriate.
4. Every four compressions, inflate the lungs once; watch the chest rise and fall with each inflation.
5. When you can, have a look at the size of the patient's pupils. Small pupils indicate effective resuscitation; fixed, dilated pupils may indicate brain damage from hypoxia. If the pupils are initially large, but then become smaller, your efforts are succeeding.
6. When help is available, set up an intravenous infusion while maintaining ventilation and massage, and give sodium bicarbonate in a dose of 1 mmol/kg of body weight (an 8.4% sodium bicarbonate solution contains 1 mmol/ml).
7. Confirm that the cardiac rhythm has been re-established, by obtaining an electrocardiogram, and treat any dysrhythmias.
8. Investigate the cause of the patient's cardiac arrest and try to determine why it happened when it did. Consider possibilities such as:
   - hypoxia
   - drug overdose
   - allergic reaction
   - myocardial infarction
   - pulmonary embolism
   - disturbance of electrolytes (especially potassium)
   - hypovolaemia.

   Treat the underlying cause of the arrest once you have identified it.
9. Consider using the following drugs in immediate management:
   - calcium gluconate for poor myocardial function and short-term protection against hyperkalaemia, up to 1 g intravenously for adults;
   - potassium for proven hypokalaemia, up to 0.3 mmol/kg of body weight given intravenously over not less than 5 min;
   - epinephrine, 0.5 mg subcutaneously for allergic reactions; 0.1–0.5 mg intravenously for asystole (confirmed by electrocardiogram, or if there is no cardiac output in spite of an acceptable heart rhythm);
   - atropine 1 mg intravenously for bradycardia;
   - lidocaine, bolus of 1 mg/kg of body weight intravenously for ventricular dysrhythmias.

If your resuscitation is successful, ensure that the patient continues to receive treatment for the underlying cause of the cardiac arrest. Maintain a safe airway after the patient starts to breathe spontaneously again. Do not remove the endotracheal tube until the patient has regained consciousness and protective reflexes.

4 Principles of fluid and electrolyte therapy

The body consists of about 60% water by weight in adults, and up to 75% in neonates. Changes in amount and composition of body fluids, which may occur as a result of bleeding, burns, dehydration, vomiting, diarrhoea, and even preoperative and postoperative starvation, can cause a severe physiological disturbance. If any such disturbance is not adequately corrected before anaesthesia and surgery, the risk to the patient is great.

Fluid compartments of the body

The body fluids can be represented as being divided into an intracellular compartment and an extracellular compartment. The extracellular compartment is further divided into intravascular and interstitial compartments (Fig. 4.1).

The intravascular compartment

Normal blood volume is about 70 ml/kg of body weight in adults and 85–90 ml/kg in neonates. In addition to the cellular components of blood, the intravascular compartment contains plasma proteins and ions, chiefly sodium (138–145 mmol/litre), chloride (97–105 mmol/litre), and bicarbonate ions. Only a small proportion of the body's potassium is present in plasma (3.5–4.5 mmol/litre), but the concentration of potassium ions is of great significance for cardiac and neuromuscular function.

The interstitial compartment

The interstitial compartment is larger than the intravascular compartment; anatomically it corresponds roughly to the interstitial spaces of the body. The total amount of extracellular fluid (intravascular plus interstitial) varies between 20% and 25% of body weight in adults and between 40% and 50% in neonates. Water and electrolytes can pass freely between the blood and the interstitial spaces, which have similar ionic composition, but plasma proteins are not free to pass out of the intravascular space unless there is damage to the capillaries, for example as a result of burns or septic shock. If there is a water deficit in the blood or a rapid fall in blood volume, water and electrolytes pass from the interstitial compartment into the blood to restore the circulating (intravascular) volume, which physiologically has priority. Intravenously administered fluids that contain mainly sodium and chloride ions, such as physiological (9 g/litre or 0.9%) saline or Hartmann's solution (Ringer's lactate solution), pass freely into the interstitial space and are therefore effective in raising the volume of intravascular fluid only for a short time. Solutions containing much larger molecules, for example plasma, whole blood, dextran, polygeline, hydroxyethyl starch, and gelatin, are more effective in maintaining the circulation when given intravenously because they remain in the intravascular compartment for a longer period. These fluids are often referred to as "plasma expanders".

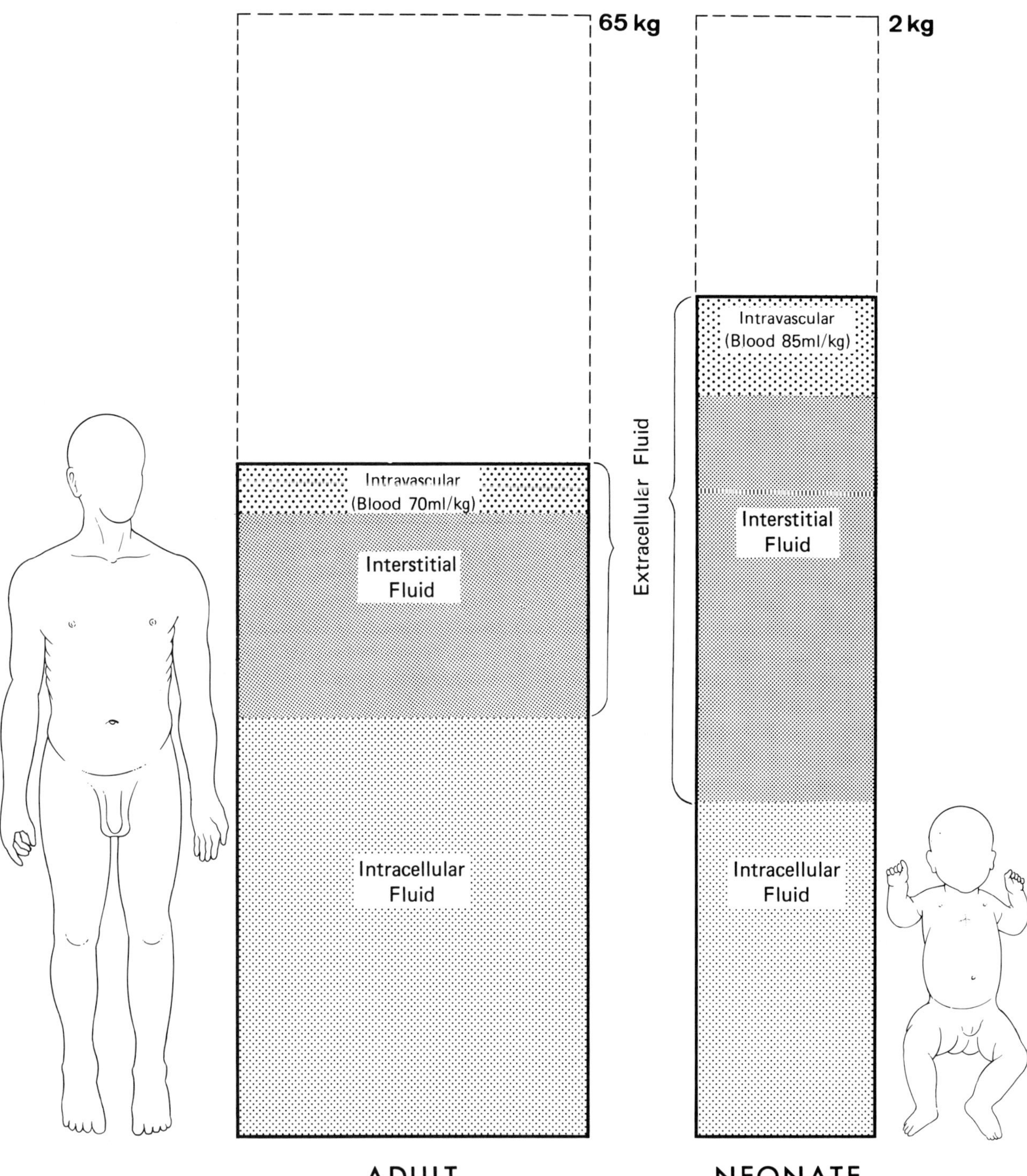

Fig. 4.1. Fluid compartments of the body.

The intracellular compartment

The intracellular compartment is the largest reservoir of body water, and corresponds to water within cells. Its ionic composition differs from that of extracellular fluid chiefly because it contains a high concentration of potassium ions (140–150 mmol/litre) and low concentrations of sodium ions (8–10 mmol/litre) and chloride ions (3 mmol/litre). Thus if water is given with sodium and chloride ions, it tends to remain in the extracellular compartment. Water given as a glucose solution can be distributed throughout all body compartments, the glucose being metabolized. Pure water must never be given intravenously, since it will immediately cause massive haemolysis.

Fluid therapy

The cardinal principle of fluid therapy is that the fluids given should be as close as possible in volume and composition to those lost. Acute losses should be replaced promptly; more caution is needed with the replacement of chronic

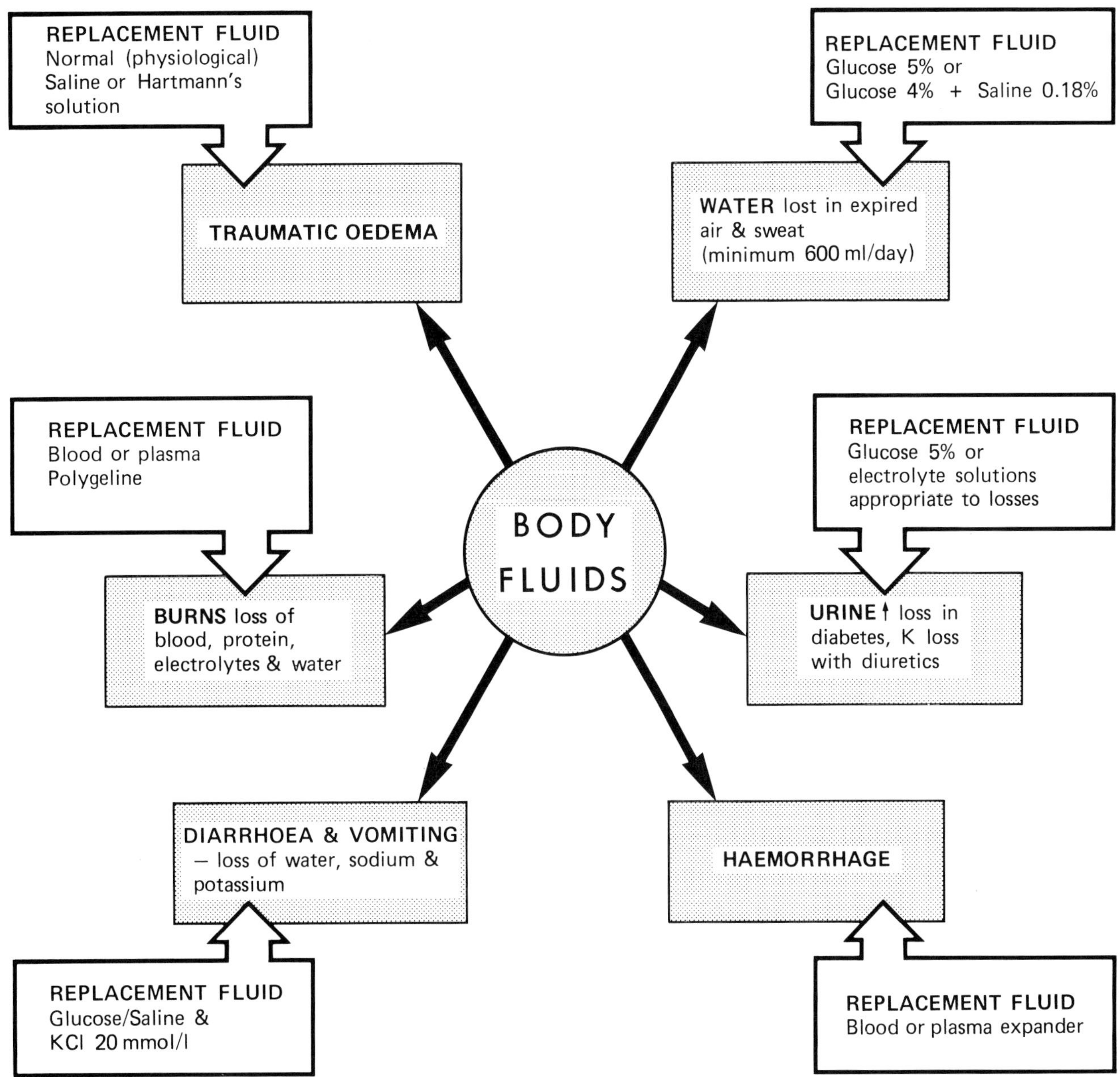

Fig. 4.2. Fluid losses and some appropriate fluids for intravenous replacement.

losses, because fast infusions into chronically malnourished and dehydrated patients can cause rapidly fatal heart failure. Chronic fluid losses are better replaced by oral or, in the absence of diarrhoea, rectal rehydration therapy. It is particularly important not to give a sodium overload to a dehydrated patient who is deficient mainly in water.

Fig. 4.2 indicates the many possible ways in which body fluid can be lost and the replacement solutions most likely to be of value for intravenous therapy. Table 1 shows the main features of commonly available replacement fluids.

Clinical assessment of fluid status

As with all clinical assessments, your task will be much easier if you first obtain an accurate history of the patient's condition, either from the patient or from a relative. This will often help you to decide which fluids have been lost, whether the loss has been acute or chronic, and what form replacement should take.

The patient's general appearance may help you assess fluid losses, though up to 10% of body water can be lost without obvious clinical signs. Greater losses cause

Table 1. Commonly available replacement fluids

Fluid	Ions (mmol/litre) Na+	Cl−	K+	Carbo-hydrate (g/litre)	Energy content (kJ [kcal$_{th}$])	Uses
Blood	140	100	4	5–8	NA	Blood loss
Physiological saline (9 g/litre)[a]	154	154	0	0	0	Blood/extracellular fluid loss
Hartmann's solution (Ringer's lactate solution)	131	112	5	NA	NA	Blood/extracellular fluid loss
Glucose 50 g/litre	0	0	0	50	837 [200]	Dehydration
Glucose/saline (glucose 40 g/litre + sodium chloride 1.8 g/litre)	31	31	0	40	669 [160]	Maintenance of electrolyte and water balance
Sodium bicarbonate 84 g/litre	1000	0	0	0	0	Acute acidosis
Dextran 70 in physiological saline	144	144	0	0	0	Intravascular replacement
Polygeline	145	150	0	0	669 [160]	Intravascular replacement

[a] The same as a 0.9% solution.
NA, not applicable.

sunken eyes, loss of tissue turgor, and a dry tongue, though these signs may be masked by oedema from hypoalbuminaemia or obesity. Cool, cyanosed extremities and invisible peripheral veins are further signs of hypovolaemia, and blood pressure may be low with an associated tachycardia. During controlled ventilation, the patient's blood pressure may fall dramatically or the pulse wave may disappear completely with each inspiratory stroke of the bellows. Urinary output may be low, and the relative density (specific gravity) of the urine high. The blood urea concentration will be higher than normal, as will the haemoglobin concentration and the erythrocyte volume fraction, unless the patient was previously anaemic. Initial investigation of the patient should include weighing — a simple and economical way of later assessing how much fluid has been replaced. A patient with severe depletion must be given fully corrective fluid therapy before anaesthesia. This applies to both general and spinal anaesthesia, as either of these can cause fatal cardiovascular collapse in volume-depleted patients. In extreme conditions, for example torrential obstetric bleeding, where surgery cannot be delayed, local infiltration of anaesthetic can be regarded as the only safe (or as the least unsafe) technique.

Estimation of blood losses during surgery

Once the patient's preoperative fluid and blood losses have been fully corrected, you should normally aim to replace intravenously any blood loss during surgery that you expect will exceed 5–10% of the patient's blood volume. For relatively small losses, clear fluids such as physiological saline may be used. If blood loss exceeds 15% of the patient's calculated blood volume, consider blood transfusion, depending on the preoperative haemoglobin level (see page 117 for further discussion of haemoglobin levels). Expertise at estimating blood loss comes with experience. Whenever possible, ask for the swabs to be weighed (before they dry out) to give you an idea of blood loss. Take the opportunity to deliberately soak a swab with 20 ml of blood to give yourself a mental picture of this volume of blood. Always use graduated suction jars; a small measuring cylinder can be used for paediatric surgery.

In addition to the blood lost during the operation — from the wound on to swabs, drapes, and the floor, and into the sucker and surgical drains — fluid is lost from the circulation and other extracellular compartments into traumatized tissue as oedema fluid. If the mesentery with an area of 1 m^2 becomes thickened with oedema by 1 mm, the fluid lost from the circulation will be 1 litre. During major surgery, it is standard practice to give clear fluids at a rate of 5 ml/kg of body weight per hour, using Hartmann's solution or physiological saline for adults and glucose 5% or glucose 4% with saline 0.18% for small children who do not have the capacity to excrete large quantities of sodium ions.

The anaesthetist is responsible for estimating blood and fluid losses in the operating theatre and for prescribing fluid replacement during and after the operation. It is best to reassess the patient constantly and not to prescribe a fluid regime for more than 6–12 hours at a time, particularly for sick patients and for children.

Specific losses and replacement

Water

Water depletion occurs most commonly because of inadequate intake (often due to illness itself) in the face of continuing or excessive losses, for example due to sweating, fever, or diarrhoea. If rehydration by the oral or rectal route is not possible, the best way to give water intravenously is as a 5% (50 g/litre) glucose solution. This solution should not be regarded as a "feeding" solution, as the carbohydrate and calorie content is low (only 837 kJ or 200 $kcal_{th}$ per litre). For patients whose condition is stable and who also require electrolyte therapy, 2–3 litres of glucose/saline solution (4% glucose, 0.18% sodium chloride) provide the average daily requirement of both water and sodium for an adult in a temperate climate.

Diarrhoea and vomiting

Diarrhoea and vomiting usually involve losses of water and of sodium, potassium, and other ions. Replacement is best done orally if possible, using a solution of oral rehydration salts (ORS)[1] or equivalent. Intravenous replacement will require saline, glucose solution (for the water it contains), and potassium. The exact proportions needed can be determined by measuring the patient's plasma electrolyte concentrations and haematological variables. It is important to avoid a sodium overload, particularly in children.

Haemorrhage and burns

The ideal replacement fluid is the one closest in composition to the one lost — blood or plasma. For initial resuscitation of the patient with hypovolaemic shock, the use of saline or Hartmann's solution is common, but you must remember that these may rapidly move out of the circulation into other compartments. Alternatively, a "plasma expander" may be used. These are natural or synthetic substances with a high relative molecular mass (molecular weight) that are retained within the blood vessels and that in turn retain fluid in the vessels because of the osmotic pressure they exert (in the same way as plasma proteins). Examples are the dextrans, polygeline, hydroxyethyl starch, and gelatin. These substances can be used in cases of severe haemorrhage to reduce the requirement for whole blood, but they cannot of course transport oxygen. For severe haemorrhage, blood transfusion is essential.

Production of sterile fluids for intravenous use

Sterile fluids for intravenous use are relatively costly. Consequently, some hospitals prepare their own supplies, if the quantities they use justify the considerable effort involved. In certain countries, for example the United Republic of Tanzania, a "do-it-yourself" production kit is available. The basic requirements for producing fluids for intravenous use are a clean and reliable water supply, availability of the appropriate chemical salts, pyrogen-free glass bottles and stoppers that can be autoclaved, an efficient autoclave, and trained staff.

[1] A solution of oral rehydration salts (ORS) contains 20 g glucose (anhydrous), 3.5 g sodium chloride, 2.9 g trisodium citrate dihydrate, and 1.5 g potassium chloride per litre.

5
Assessing the patient before anaesthesia

Failure to make a proper assessment of the patient's condition is one of the commonest and most easily avoidable causes of mishaps associated with anaesthesia. There is no such thing as a "minor" anaesthetic, and all patients need to be properly assessed before anaesthesia by the person who will administer the anaesthetic. Such an assessment must include every aspect of the patient's condition, and not just the pathological problem requiring surgery.

The initial assessment of a patient includes taking a full medical history; certain points will be of particular interest to the anaesthetist. The pathological problem requiring surgery and the operation proposed are also of obvious importance, and you will want to know how long the procedure is likely to take. Ask the patient about previous operations and anaesthetics and about any serious medical illnesses in the past, with specific inquiry about malaria, jaundice, haemoglobinopathies, and diseases of the cardiovascular or respiratory systems. In relation to the patient's current health, ask about exercise tolerance, cough, dyspnoea, wheeze, chest pains, dizzy spells, and blackouts. Is the patient taking any regular drug therapy? Drugs of special significance to anaesthesia include antidiabetic drugs, anticoagulants, antibiotics, steroids, and antihypertensive drugs — treatment with the last two should be maintained during anaesthesia and surgery, but other types of drug therapy should be modified as necessary. Note any known allergies on the drug prescription chart (you cannot wake the patient up during the operation to check!) together with any known adverse reactions to anaesthesia experienced in the past by either the patient or the patient's blood-relations. (The dangerous conditions of suxamethonium apnoea and malignant hyperthermia are often familial, so any patient with a family history of such conditions should be referred to a larger hospital. In an emergency it would probably be safe to anaesthetize the patient with ketamine or a local anaesthetic, but suxamethonium is absolutely contraindicated.)

Finally, assess recent fluid losses from bleeding, vomiting, diarrhoea, or other causes and ask about the patient's dietary history. Has he or she been able to eat and drink normally up to the time of admission? If not, you should suspect fluid or nutritional deficiences and take active steps to correct these before the operation. Find out when the patient last had any food or drink, and explain the need for fasting before anaesthesia.

Examining the patient

Look first for general signs of illness. Is your patient pale, jaundiced, cyanosed, dehydrated, malnourished, oedematous, dyspnoeic, or in pain?

Next take a good look at the patient's upper airway and consider how you are going to manage it during anaesthesia. Will the airway become obstructed easily? Will it be easy or difficult to intubate? (Most are easy!) Has the patient any loose or awkward teeth or a small lower jaw, which will make laryngoscopy difficult? Is there any restriction to mouth opening or any stiffness of the neck? Are there any abnormal swellings in the neck that could distort the anatomy of the upper airway? *Now is the time to find out.*

Examine the patient for evidence of cardiac or respiratory disease, and in particular for cardiac valvular disease (for which prophylactic antibiotics will be required to protect the patient during surgery), hypertension (look at the optic fundi), and left-sided or right-sided cardiac failure with elevated venous pressure, ankle or sacral oedema, hepatic enlargement, or basal crepitations. Look at the shape of the chest and the activity of the respiratory muscles for evidence of acute or chronic airway obstruction or respiratory failure. Palpate the trachea to see if it is displaced by fibrosis, by the collapse of all or part of a lung, or by pneumothorax. Percuss the chest wall for areas of dullness that may be due to the collapse of a lung or effusion. Listen for wheezing or râles, which may indicate generalized or localized bronchial obstruction.

The abdomen also deserves your attention. Enlargement of the liver may point to disease caused by a high alcohol intake or to other forms of liver disease that can affect the patient's response to anaesthetic drugs. (A cirrhotic liver is usually shrunken and impalpable.) If you are in a part of the world where malaria is prevalent, check the patient's spleen; hypersplenism can lead to problems in blood coagulation. Distension of the abdomen by intestinal gas, ascites, an abdominal tumour, or even a gravid uterus can cause severe respiratory embarrassment when the patient lies down. (Obstetric anaesthesia, which has special problems and requires special consideration, is dealt with in Chapter 13.)

At this stage in the examination you may have diagnosed several problems in addition to the one that requires surgery. Decide whether further investigations (for example laboratory tests, X-ray examination, and electrocardiography) are needed. A routine X-ray examination of the patient's chest is not necessary if there are no abnormal symptoms or signs referable to the chest, but measurement of haemoglobin concentration or erythrocyte volume fraction should be routine if the patient is having a general anaesthetic or anything other than a minor operation under conduction anaesthesia.

When all the results are available, ask yourself three further questions:

1. Can the patient's condition be further improved by preoperative treatment?
2. Should the patient be referred for treatment of underlying conditions, for example anaemia, infections, or dietary deficiency, before surgery?
3. What anaesthetic technique is most suitable for the patient? (See Chapter 11.)

When you have decided on your anaesthetic technique, explain briefly to the patient what will happen, with reassurance that you will be present all the time to look after breathing and the function of the heart and to make sure that he or she feels no pain. Also tell the patient what to expect on awakening, for example oxygen, an intravenous infusion, a nasogastric tube, or surgical drains. A few minutes of explanation and kindness in your approach will relieve many of the patient's anxieties and make your task as anaesthetist much easier.

Finally, prescribe any premedication you wish the patient to have (see below).

In making a simple and efficient preoperative assessment, you may find a check-list (as shown in Fig. 5.1) helpful. A single chart could combine a preoperative check-list, an anaesthetic chart (as in Annex 3), and a postoperative instruction sheet.

Preoperative Check-list

Part 1

Hospital no. ....
Surname ....
First name ....

Date ....
Ward ....
Blood group ....

History

SERIOUS ILLNESSES
- Cardiovascular ....
- Respiratory ....
- Other systemic ....
- Diabetes ....
- Haemoglobinopathies ....

CURRENT HEALTH ....

CURRENT/RECENT DRUGS
- Corticosteroids ....
- Anticoagulants ....
- Antibiotics ....
- Antihypertensives ....
- Antidiabetics ....

ALLERGIES ....

ADVERSE REACTION TO PREVIOUS ANAESTHETIC (SELF/RELATIVE) ....

RECENT FLUID LOSSES
- Bleeding ....
- Vomiting ....
- Diarrhoea ....
- Other ....

RECENT NUTRITION
- Food: normal/abnormal
- Fluids: normal/abnormal

DATE OF LAST MENSTRUAL PERIOD ....

Fig. 5.1. Preoperative check-list.

Preoperative Check-list

Part 2

Physical examination

GENERAL CONDITION

Conjunctivae ....
Anaemia ....
Hydration ....
Teeth ....
Cyanosis ....

UPPER AIRWAYS

Obstruction: likely/unlikely
Intubation: probably simple/difficult

RESPIRATORY SYSTEM

Cough .... Dyspnoea ....
Wheeze .... Sputum ....

SHAPE OF CHEST

Normal expansion .... Percussion ....

FINDINGS ON AUSCULTATION ....

CARDIOVASCULAR SYSTEM

Heart rate ....
regular/irregular
Blood pressure ....
Precordium
Left ventricle: normal/enlarged
Right ventricle: normal/enlarged
Thrills ....
Murmurs ....
Functional diagnosis ....
Signs of cardiac failure ....

ABDOMEN

Thin/obese
Distension ....
Ascites ....

Further investigations ordered & results

Premedication for anaesthesia and surgery

A patient about to undergo surgery is usually given premedication for one or more of the following reasons:

- to provide sedation and relieve anxiety associated with fear of the unknown (although this is unnecessary in children under 2 years old);
- to provide sedation to make it easier to use conduction anaesthesia;
- to provide analgesia if the patient has pain before the operation or to provide a background of analgesia during and after the operation;
- to suppress secretions, especially before the use of ether or ketamine (the drying agent atropine is given for this purpose and may also be used to block vagal activity and prevent bradycardia, especially in children);
- to reduce the risk of aspiration of acid gastric contents if gastric emptying is impaired, for example in pregnancy (in such cases antacids are given orally).

Drugs for premedication should be given in a dose related to the patient's weight and general condition. The normal routes for premedication are intramuscularly 1 hour or orally 2 hours before anaesthesia.

Many anaesthetists prefer to avoid heavy opiate premedication if anaesthesia is to include spontaneous respiration of ether/air mixtures. The following drugs are widely used:

Opiate analgesics	morphine 0.15 mg/kg intramuscularly pethidine 1.0 mg/kg intramuscularly	
Sedatives	diazepam 0.15 mg/kg orally or intramuscularly pentobarbital 3 mg/kg orally or 1.5 mg/kg intramuscularly	adults
	promethazine 0.5 mg/kg orally chloral hydrate syrup 30 mg/kg	children
Vagolytic antisialogogue	atropine 0.02 mg/kg intramuscularly or intravenously at induction, maximum 0.5 mg	
Antacids	sodium citrate 0.3 mol/litre aluminium hydroxide suspension	10–20 ml

6
General anaesthesia

Inhalational anaesthesia forms the basis of most general anaesthetic techniques in common use, although intravenous techniques are an alternative. There are two different systems available to deliver anaesthetic gases and vapours to the patient. In the draw-over system, air is used as the carrier gas to which volatile agents or compressed medical gases are added. In the continuous-flow system air is not used, but compressed medical gases, usually nitrous oxide and oxygen, pass through flow meters (rotameters) and vaporizers to supply anaesthetic to the patient.

Continuous-flow anaesthetic machines (usually known as Boyle's machines) can be used only if there is a guaranteed supply of oxygen and preferably of nitrous oxide also. These gases are not always easy to obtain, and nitrous oxide is relatively expensive. A potential hazard in using compressed gases is that, should the oxygen supply run out during anaesthesia, the machine may continue to deliver nitrous oxide alone, and this will rapidly kill the patient. Various alarms and interlock devices have been fitted to Boyle's machines to minimize this risk, but none is fully satisfactory. A draw-over system, which is open to the atmosphere at one end, cannot deliver substantially less than the atmospheric concentration of oxygen, which is 20.9% by volume, and can be used even if no cylinders of gas are available. In many cases supplementation of the inspired gases with oxygen is desirable, and this is easily and very economically done with a draw-over system.

The draw-over system is capable of producing first-class anaesthetic and surgical conditions. In contrast to continuous-flow systems, which were first used around 1912, the modern draw-over apparatus developed in the 1940s and 1950s has proved extremely reliable, easy to understand and maintain, and economical in use. It should be the first choice for inhalational anaesthesia in all small hospitals and should be one of a variety of techniques in regular use in teaching hospitals. However, some small hospitals and many larger ones already possess continuous-flow machines, and a description of their use is therefore included in this chapter. Further development of compressors and oxygen concentrators (see page 126) may in the future allow the use of Boyle's machines without supplies of compressed medical gas, but at present no machine of this type exists that would be suitable for use in small hospitals.

The state of anaesthesia can be produced by several different types of drug with differing properties. The aim is to provide a pleasant induction and lack of awareness for the patient, using a technique that is safe for both patient and anaesthetist and that provides good operating conditions for the surgeon. Unfortunately, the ideal anaesthetic drug with all the desired qualities does not exist. It is common practice, therefore, to combine several drugs, each of which provides a single "component" of anaesthesia. This can be represented diagrammatically as a triangle whose corners represent sleep (unconsciousness), muscular relaxation, and analgesia (lack of response to painful stimulation) (Fig. 6.1).

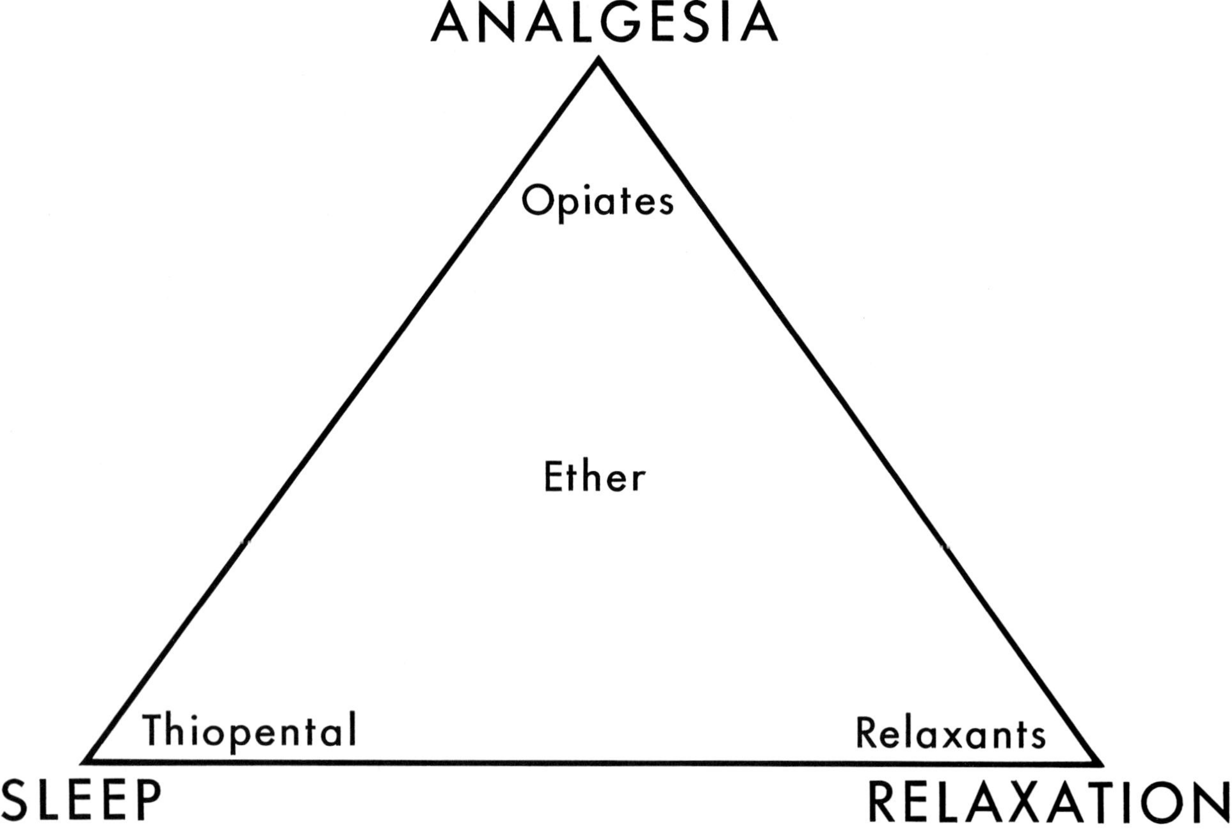

Fig. 6.1. Balanced anaesthesia represented as a triangle.

Certain drugs, for example thiopental, produce sleep without relaxation or analgesia, which makes them suitable for use only for inducing anaesthesia. In contrast, ether produces a mixture of sleep, analgesia, and relaxation, but because of its pungent smell and high solubility in blood it is rather inconvenient and slow (though safe) for induction of anaesthesia. The muscle relaxants produce muscular relaxation alone, and may therefore be used to provide good surgical relaxation during light anaesthesia, which allows the patient to recover rapidly at the end of anaesthesia. Opiate drugs like morphine and pethidine produce analgesia with little change in muscle tone or level of consciousness. Several combinations of techniques and drugs are available, and the choice of the most suitable combination for any given patient and operation calls for careful thought and planning.

Before induction of anaesthesia

Anaesthesia is often compared to flying an aeroplane — most crashes happen during take-off and landing — so special care is needed during induction and recovery.

Before starting, check that you have the correct patient scheduled for the correct operation on the correct side. The responsibility for this check belongs to both anaesthetist and surgeon. Check that the patient has been properly prepared for the operation and has had no food or drink for at least 6 hours, though milk-fed babies need be starved for only 3 hours. (For induction of anaesthesia for emergency surgery when the patient possibly has a full stomach, see page 77.) Measure the patient's pulse and blood pressure, and try to make him or her as relaxed and comfortable as possible. Make sure that an experienced and trained assistant is available to help you with induction. *Under no circumstances should you induce anaesthesia when alone with the patient.*

Checking your equipment

It is vital to check your equipment before you give an anaesthetic; indeed, the patient's life may depend on it. You should have copied out the appropriate check-list from Annexes 1 and 2 and hung it permanently on any anaesthetic apparatus you may use.

First make sure that all the apparatus you intend to use or might need is actually available. If you are using compressed gases, check the pressure in the cylinders in use and also in the reserve cylinders. Check that the anaesthetic vaporizers are connected properly with no leaks and no loose or missing filling caps and that the breathing system that delivers gas to the patient is securely and correctly assembled. If you are at all uncertain about the breathing system, try breathing through it yourself (with the supply of anaesthetic agents turned off). Check the functioning of the resuscitation apparatus (which must always be present in case of a gas supply failure), the laryngoscope, the endotracheal tubes (by inflating the cuff to check for leaks), and the suction apparatus. You must also ensure that anaesthesia is induced with the patient lying on a table or trolley that can be rapidly tilted into a head-down position to cope with possible sudden hypotension or vomiting.

Draw up the drugs you intend to use into labelled syringes and make sure that any drugs you might need are actually available.

Before inducing anaesthesia, ensure adequate intravenous access by inserting an indwelling needle or cannula into a large vein; for major surgery an intravenous infusion of an appropriate fluid should be started immediately.

The choice of technique for induction of anaesthesia lies between:

- intravenous injection of a barbiturate or ketamine
- intramuscular injection of ketamine
- inhalational induction.

Intravenous induction

This is pleasant for the patient and easy for the anaesthetist. It will be the technique of choice in many cases, but care is always needed, as it is relatively easy to give an overdose or to stop the patient from breathing. If breathing stops, the patient may die unless you can easily ventilate the lungs with a face mask or endotracheal tube. The first rule of intravenous induction is that it must *never* be used in a patient whose airway is likely to be difficult to manage. For such a patient inhalational induction is inherently much safer, or the patient should be intubated while still awake.

Induction with a barbiturate (see also page 82)

The barbiturate thiopental is presented as ampoules of yellow powder that must be dissolved before use in sterile distilled water or saline to make a solution of 2.5% (25 mg/ml). Higher concentrations are dangerous, especially if accidentally injected outside a vein, and should not be used. The normal practice is to give a "sleep" dose by injecting the drug slowly until the patient becomes unconscious and loses the eyelash reflex. The average sleep dose in a healthy adult is 4–5 mg/kg of body weight, but in sick patients much less is needed. An overdose of thiopental will cause hypotension by depressing the vasomotor centre and respiratory arrest by depressing the respiratory centre.

Injection of thiopental is almost always painless. If the patient reports pain, stop injecting immediately, because the needle is probably outside the vein and may even have entered an artery. (Avoid injection into the cubital fossa, if possible, because of the close proximity of the artery and vein.) If the point of the needle has entered an artery, leave it there and, for an adult patient, inject into the artery 5 ml of 1% lidocaine, 100 mg of hydrocortisone, and 1000 International Units of heparin to prevent arterial thrombosis; then remove the needle and infiltrate a further 5 ml of lidocaine around the artery.

Methohexital can be used as an alternative to thiopental. It also comes as a powder and should be made up as a 1% solution (10 mg/ml). The average sleep dose is around 1 mg/kg of body weight. Patients are slightly more likely to complain of pain during injection, even with a correctly placed needle, though the pain is not usually severe. The incidence of pain is higher when small veins on the back of the hand are used.

Once the patient loses consciousness stop injecting the barbiturate drug. In old or sick patients, the circulation time from arm to brain is slow, so give the drug more slowly to avoid an overdose. After induction the responsibility for protecting the patient's airway and breathing is yours. In most cases, you will want to protect the airway by inserting an endotracheal tube.

Induction with ketamine (see also page 82)

Induction with ketamine is similar in principle to induction with thiopental, and the same precautions apply. The average induction dose is 1–2 mg/kg of body weight. (The standard formulations are 50 mg/ml and 100 mg/ml, but be sure to check which one you have.) The patient's appearance as he or she loses consciousness is different from when barbiturates are used, and the patient may not appear to be "asleep". The eyes may remain open, but the patient will no longer respond to your voice or command or to painful stimuli. If you try to insert an oropharyngeal airway at this stage the patient will probably spit it out. Muscle tone in the jaw is usually well maintained after ketamine has been given, as is the cough reflex. A safe airway is not guaranteed, since if regurgitation or vomiting of gastric contents occurs, there is still severe danger of aspiration into the lungs.

After induction with ketamine, you may choose to proceed to a conventional inhalational anaesthetic, with or without relaxants and intubation. For short procedures, increments of ketamine may be given intravenously or intramuscularly every few minutes to prevent the patient responding to painful stimulation. This method of anaesthesia is simple, but produces no muscular relaxation, and ketamine is not a cheap drug. If your supplies are limited, try to reserve ketamine for cases where there are few suitable alternatives, for example for short procedures in children when access to the airway may be difficult.

Intramuscular induction

Ketamine may also be given by intramuscular injection to induce anaesthesia. With a dose of 6–8 mg/kg of body weight, induction occurs within a few minutes, followed by 10–15 min of surgical anaesthesia. At 8 mg/kg, ketamine produces a marked increase in salivary secretions, necessitating injection of atropine (which can be mixed with the ketamine). Subsequent increments of ketamine can be given intramuscularly or intravenously, as required. Intramuscular doses last longer and wear off more slowly. If ketamine is used as the sole anaesthetic agent, patients sometimes complain afterwards of vivid dreams and hallucinations. The incidence of such hallucinations can be reduced by giving diazepam either before or at the end of anaesthesia. Hallucinations do not occur if ketamine is used only for induction and is followed by a conventional anaesthetic.

Inhalational induction

This is the technique of choice for inducing anaesthesia when the patient's airway is difficult to manage. If you use an intravenous induction for such a patient and "lose" the airway, the patient may die of hypoxia if you are unable to ventilate the lungs. In contrast, inhalational induction can proceed only if the patient has a clear airway down which the anaesthetic can pass. If the airway becomes obstructed, the patient will stop taking up further anaesthetic and redistribution of the drug in the body will lighten the anaesthesia. As this happens the patient will clear the obstruction. Inhalational induction is also preferred by some children, who may object to needles.

Inhalational induction is an important technique and should be practised regularly; despite the many points to be considered, it is simple and requires only patience, care, and observation. Either draw-over or continuous-flow apparatus can be used for inhalational induction (Fig. 6.2), but slightly differing techniques are needed.

Induction using draw-over apparatus

The recommended agents for inhalational induction with draw-over apparatus are ether (for example from the EMO, Afya, or PAC vaporizer), halothane, and trichloroethylene (both from, for example, the PAC or Oxford Miniature Vaporizer). If oxygen is available, it should be added with a T-piece, as shown in Fig. 7.9, page 68. The draw-over apparatus and breathing system are assembled as shown in Fig. 7.7, page 65. If halothane or trichloroethylene is in use, the vaporizer should be downstream from the ether vaporizer.

The smoothest induction is effected by applying a well-fitting face mask gently and beginning induction with halothane (which is preferable) or trichloroethylene. Gradually increase the concentration, say by 0.5% every five breaths, until the patient is asleep (maximum 2–3% halothane or 1.5% trichloroethylene). Then slowly turn on the supply of ether and increase the concentration by 1% every five breaths. The respiratory stimulant effect of ether will increase the uptake of both itself and the halothane or trichlorethylene. If the patient coughs or holds his or her breath, reduce the ether concentration immediately by a third of its setting and try again. When you reach 8% ether, stop giving the other agent. You may then proceed to laryngoscopy and intubation after further deepening the anaesthesia by increasing the ether concentration to about 15%. Watch for the onset of paralysis of the lower intercostal muscles to show that the anaesthesia is deep enough. The addition of oxygen is desirable at least until intubation has been achieved. If your attempt at intubation does not succeed, reapply the face mask and deepen the anaesthesia again for a second attempt. If intubation is still impossible, *but* you can maintain a clear airway using a face mask, you may proceed to give anaesthetic with the face mask, using ether at 7–10% to provide relaxation if required. If relaxation is not required, reduce the ether concentration to 6%. With ether at this concentration your patient can, if necessary, manage without oxygen supplementation, provided that he or she is not very young, very old, very ill, or anaemic.

Take special care if halothane and trichloroethylene are used together as alternatives to ether, as they both depress the heart and respiration. Additional oxygen should be given if at all possible and, if not contraindicated by an airway that is difficult to manage, a muscle relaxant should be used for intubation. If oxygen is not available to supplement the halothane/trichloroethylene mixture, controlled ventilation (IPPV) should be used.

Induction using a Boyle's machine

First check your machine, making sure that you have adequate supplies of gas for the duration of anaesthesia (see check-list in Annex 2). Oxygen should be used at a concentration of not less than 30% to allow for any inaccuracy of the rotameters. If you are using nitrous oxide, set the gas flows on the rotameters to 3 litres/min of oxygen and 6 litres/min of nitrous oxide if you are using a one-way breathing valve. With a Magill breathing system, these flows may be reduced to 2 litres/min of oxygen and 4 litres/min of nitrous oxide. If you are using halothane

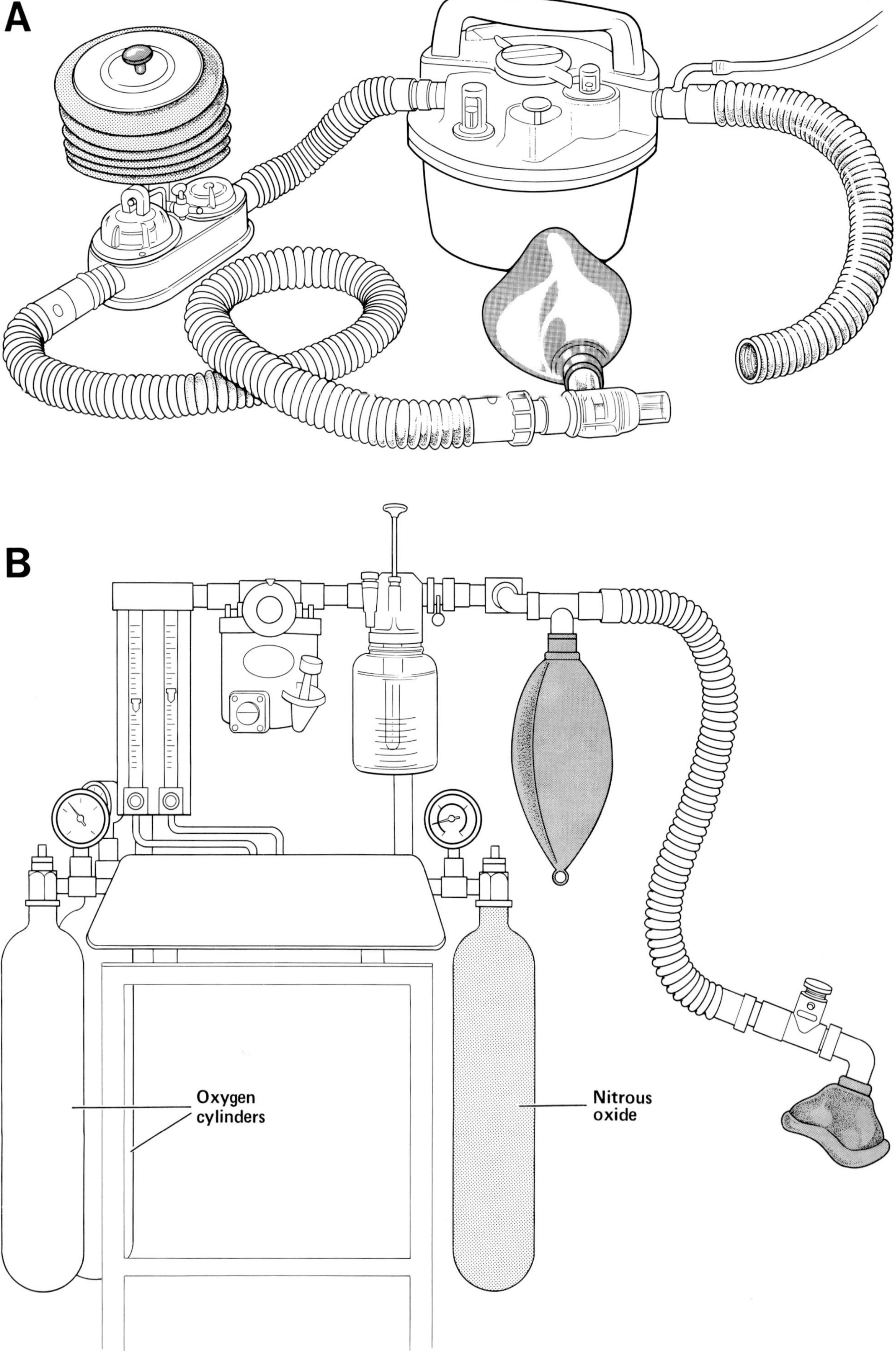

Fig. 6.2. Apparatus for inhalational anaesthesia. (A) Draw-over system; (B) continuous-flow (Boyle's) anaesthetic machine.

as your main volatile agent, place the face mask on the patient's face and gradually increase the halothane concentration up to a maximum of 3%, reducing it to 1.5% after the patient has settled or after intubation. If you are using ether (without halothane) as your volatile agent, it is easier to turn on the supply of ether from the Boyle's bottle with the face mask held about 30 cm above the patient's face. Gradually lowering the mask over the next minute will slowly increase the ether concentration in the inspired gas and is usually well tolerated. Once the mask is in contact with the face, slowly increase the ether concentration over a few minutes. The patient will be ready for intubation with the onset of paralysis of the intercostal muscles.

7
Apparatus used for inhalational anaesthesia[1]

Draw-over apparatus

Two fundamental pieces of equipment are needed for draw-over inhalational anaesthesia: a vaporizing device for the anaesthetic and a self-inflating bag or bellows (SIB) to ventilate the patient's lungs. These must be linked together and to the patient by a breathing system containing one or more one-way valves (to prevent the patient from breathing out through the vaporizer). The breathing system must connect to the patient's airway at its outlet via a breathing valve and face mask or endotracheal tube, and the inlet to the system must be open to the atmosphere to allow air to be drawn in, either by the patient's inspiratory effort or by the recoil of the SIB. Various types of apparatus are commercially available for draw-over use; some examples are shown in Fig. 7.1.

Vaporizers

For effective and safe use in a draw-over system, a vaporizer must have a low resistance to gas flow (since air must be drawn through it by the patient's inspiration), and it must be capable of accurately delivering the required concentration of vapour despite the wide fluctuations in flow that occur during the inspiratory period. The range of vaporizers currently in use includes the EMO (Epstein, Macintosh, Oxford), OMV (Oxford Miniature Vaporizer), Afya, and PAC series (Figs. 7.2 & 7.3). The OMV and EMO have a wide application, as they can also be used with continuous-flow anaesthetic systems. Vaporizers with a high internal resistance (for example the "Tec" series, Boyle's bottle, and Dräger Vapor) are completely unsuitable for draw-over use and must never be used for draw-over anaesthesia, as the patient cannot breathe through them.

When a volatile anaesthetic liquid is vaporized, heat is lost as latent heat of vaporization. If this heat loss is not compensated for, the vaporizer and contents will cool, which will result in a rapid fall-off of the concentration of vapour delivered, since the vapour pressure of the anaesthetic falls with temperature. To prevent this from occurring or to minimize its effects, most draw-over vaporizers have a thermal compensation or buffering system or both. Thermal buffering is the provision in the vaporizer of a mass of substance of high specific heat capacity (usually copper or water) that resists sudden changes in temperature. Thermo-compensation is achieved by building into the design of the vaporizer a thermostatically operated valve to control the amount of air entering the vaporizing chamber and keep constant the concentration of vapour delivered. The EMO

[1]In some cases, the apparatus described in this chapter (and elsewhere in the book) has been identified by the manufacturer's name or trademark. However, this does not imply that such products are endorsed or recommended by WHO or the author in preference to others of a similar nature that are not mentioned. Rather, the specific products mentioned represent those that are known to the author to be in common use in district hospitals with limited resources. In the event that there are others in common use, WHO would be pleased to be so informed for the purpose of including a description of their use in future editions of this book.

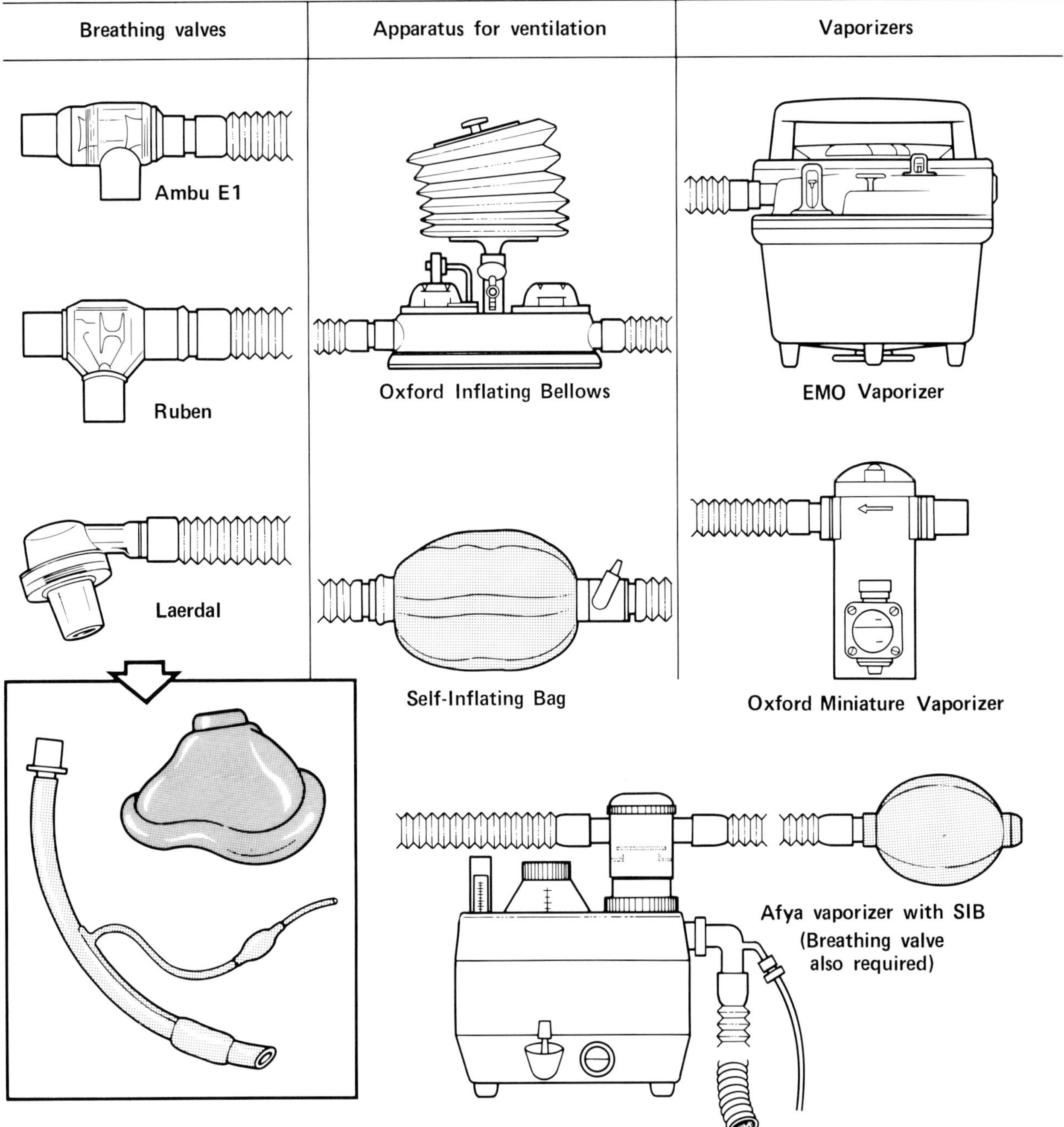

Fig. 7.1. Draw-over anaesthesia systems.

and Afya ether vaporizers use both thermocompensation and thermal buffering, with water as the heat reservoir. (New vaporizers are sent from the factory with the water chamber empty, and the first user must fill the water chamber in accordance with the manufacturer's instructions.) The thermocompensation valve of the EMO is automatic and can be seen through a small window on top of the vaporizer, which also indicates whether the vaporizer is within its thermal working range of 10–30 °C (Fig. 7.4). In normal use a black ring should show at the window. If the vaporizer overheats, for example by being left in direct sun on a hot day, a red ring also appears, and the vaporizer must be cooled before use. If the vaporizer becomes too cold, for example by being left in an aircraft luggage bay, the black ring disappears, and only an aluminium disc is visible; the vaporizer must then be allowed to warm up before use. If the black ring is not showing and the vaporizer does not appear cold, the thermocompensation valve (TC valve) may have fractured and need replacement (normal valve life is about 10 years). Replacement is relatively simple and does not require return of the vaporizer to the manufacturer.

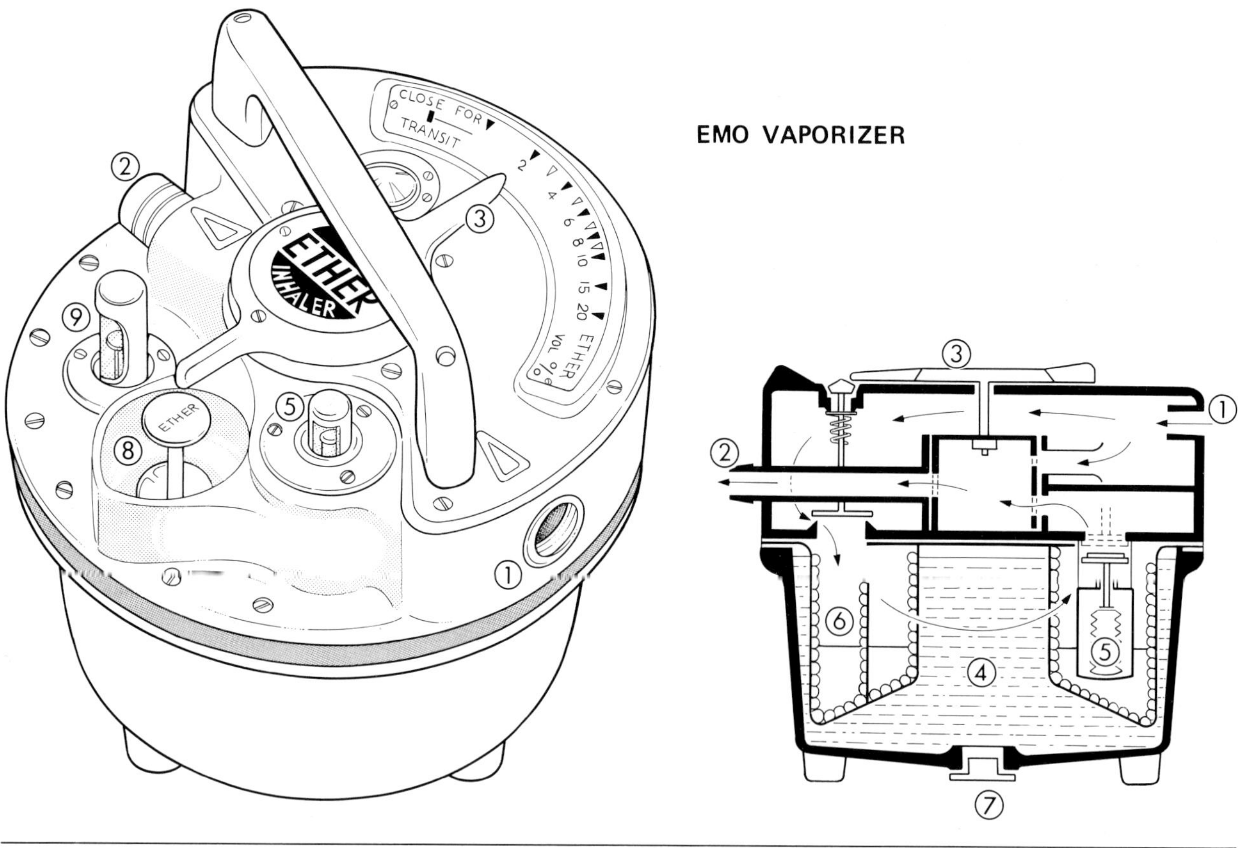

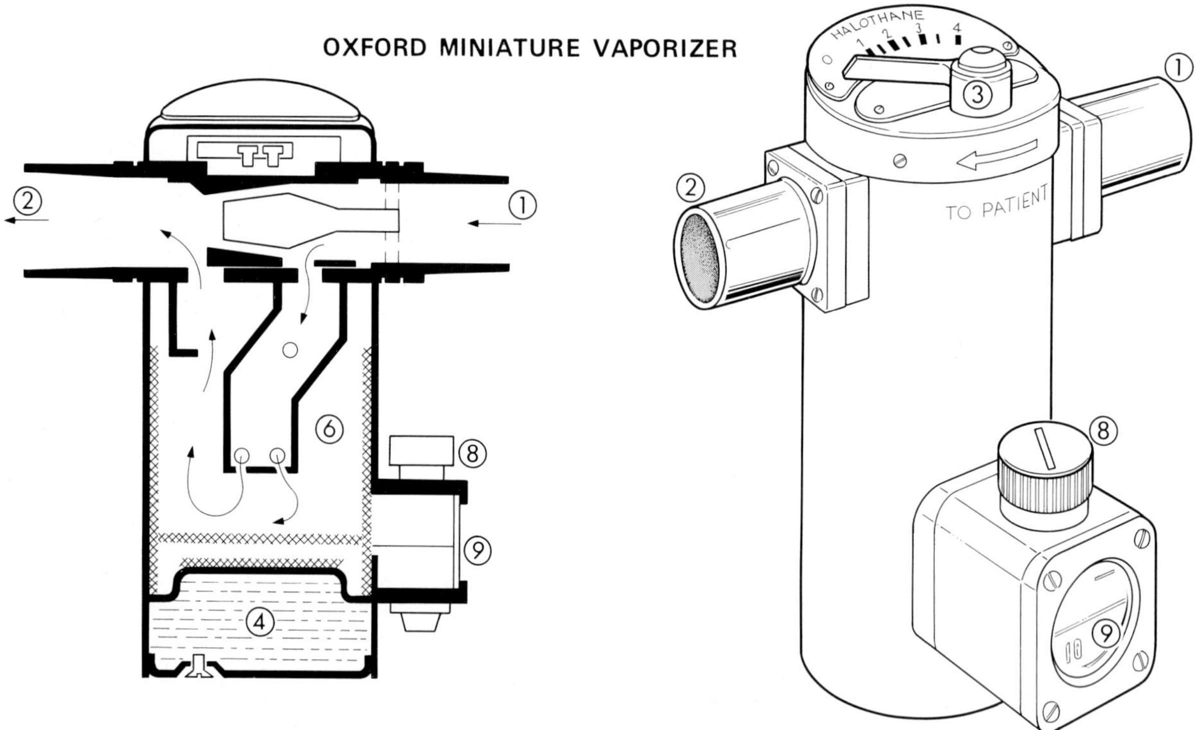

Fig. 7.2. Draw-over vaporizers (EMO and OMV). (1) Inlet port, (2) outlet port, (3) concentration control, (4) water jacket, (5) thermocompensator valve, (6) vaporizing chamber, (7) filling port for water, (8) filling port for anaesthetic, (9) anaesthetic-level indicator.

Thermocompensation of the Afya vaporizer must be controlled manually by turning a knob to indicate on a scale the temperature of the ether. A thermometer is built into the vaporizer (Fig. 7.3). The PAC series vaporizers use automatic thermocompensation and, if their accuracy is to be ensured, should be serviced only by a manufacturer's agent. The OMV does not have full thermocompensation, but changes in temperature are minimized by thermal buffering with a

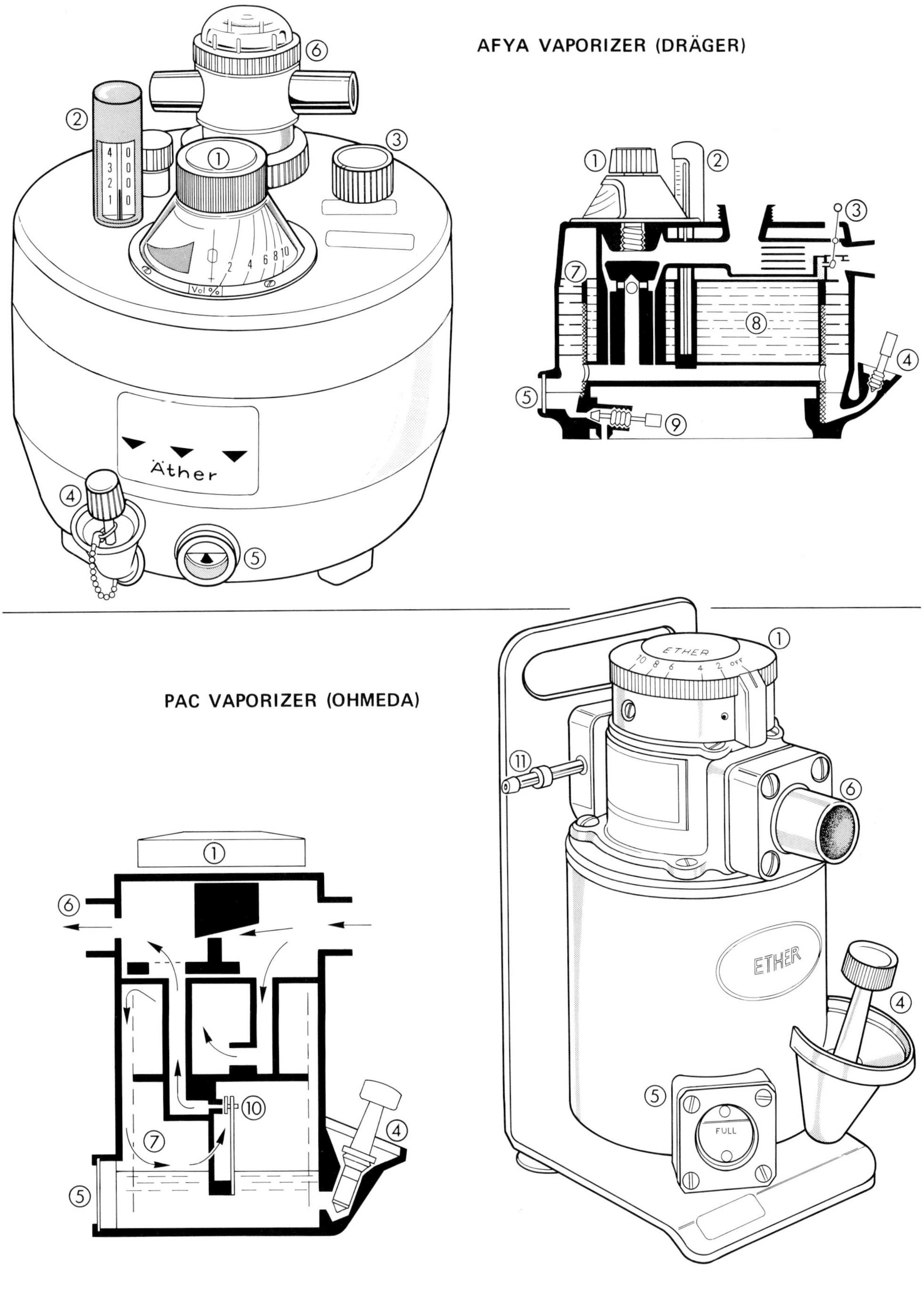

AFYA VAPORIZER (DRÄGER)

PAC VAPORIZER (OHMEDA)

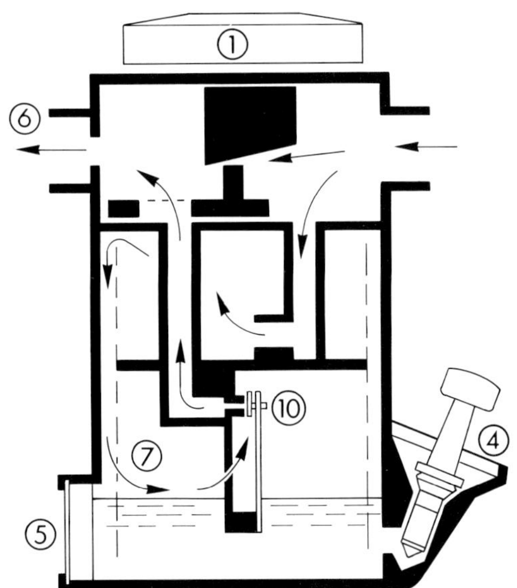

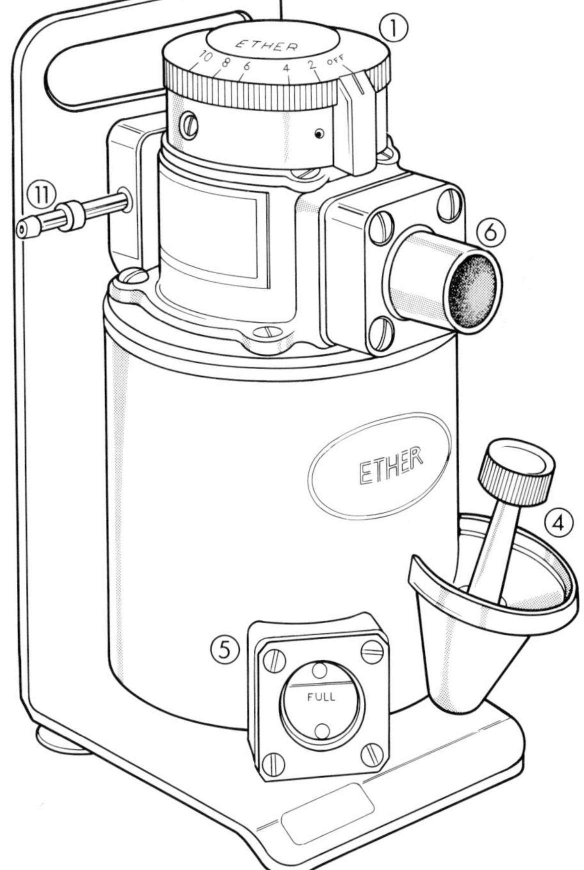

Fig. 7.3. Draw-over vaporizers (Afya and PAC). (1) Concentration control, (2) thermometer, (3) on/off control, (4) filling port for ether, (5) ether-level gauge, (6) outlet and one-way valve, (7) vaporizing chamber, (8) water-filled heat reservoir, (9) drainage port for ether, (10) thermocompensator valve, (11) port for oxygen enrichment.

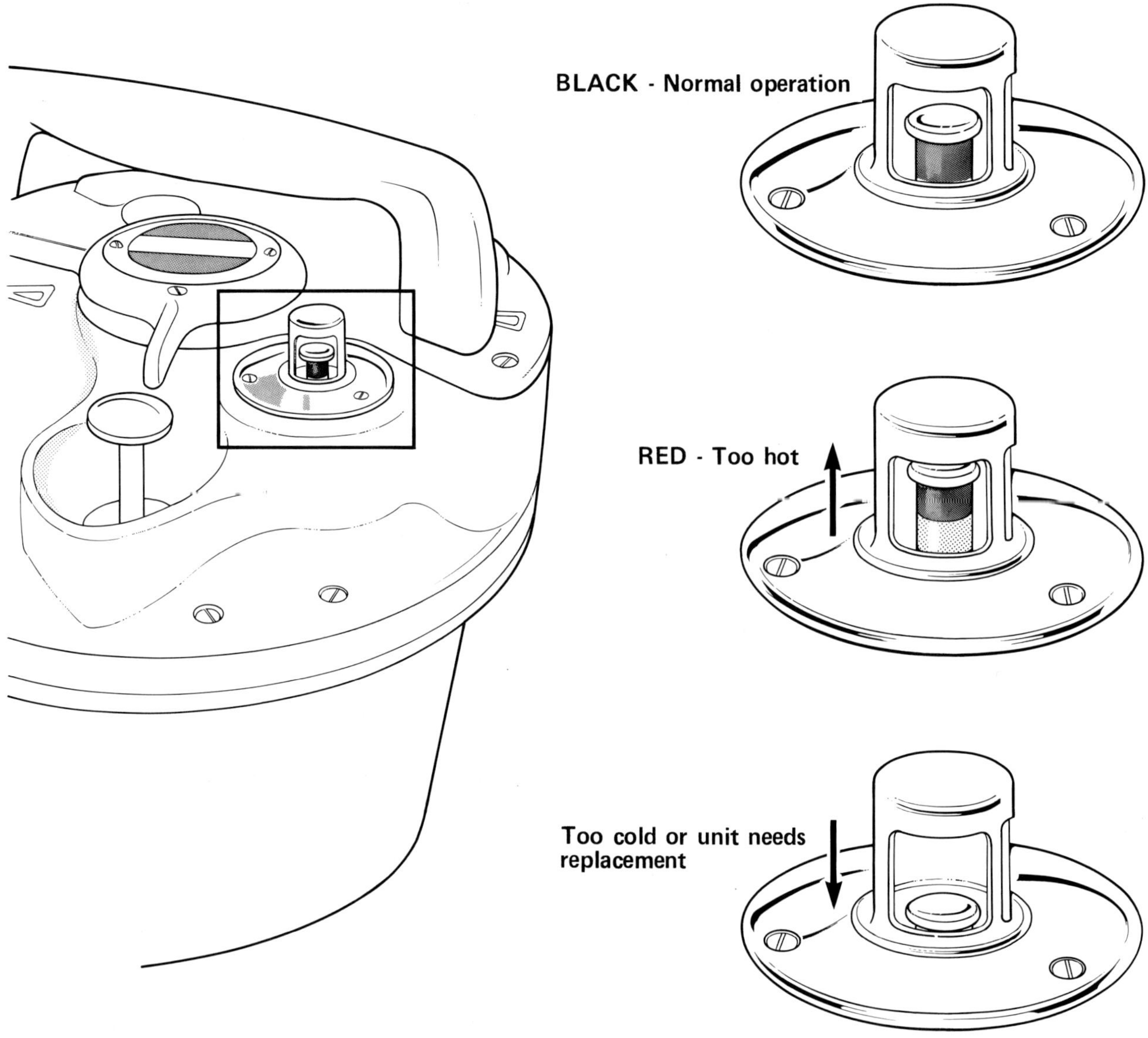

Fig. 7.4. Thermocompensation valve and temperature indicator on the EMO vaporizer.

mixture of water and antifreeze, which is put into the core of the vaporizer during manufacture and needs no further attention from the user. The output concentrations of the vaporizer are controlled with a pointer that moves over a graduated scale.

It is possible to connect two vaporizers in series, but *never* connect any vaporizer containing halothane to the *inlet* port of the EMO, since if halothane enters the EMO it rapidly causes severe corrosion. It is perfectly safe to connect a halothane vaporizer such as an OMV to the outlet port of the EMO (Fig. 7.5). In fact, the OMV was designed to be used in this position.

During anaesthesia, it may become necessary to refill the vaporizer with anaesthetic liquid. You must first turn the concentration control to the zero position before opening the filling port. If you fail to do so, air will be drawn into the vaporizing chamber and a dangerously high concentration of anaesthetic will be delivered to the patient. For the same reason, you must never use a vaporizer that has no filling plug or that has any route through which air can enter accidentally, for example a broken glass window on the filling gauge.

Breathing systems — and an important note about valves

The purpose of the breathing system (formerly called the breathing circuit) is to deliver anaesthetic vapour from the vaporizer to the patient, to pass the patient's expired gas into the atmosphere, and to provide a method of giving controlled ventilation (IPPV) when muscle relaxants are in use or for resuscitation. The

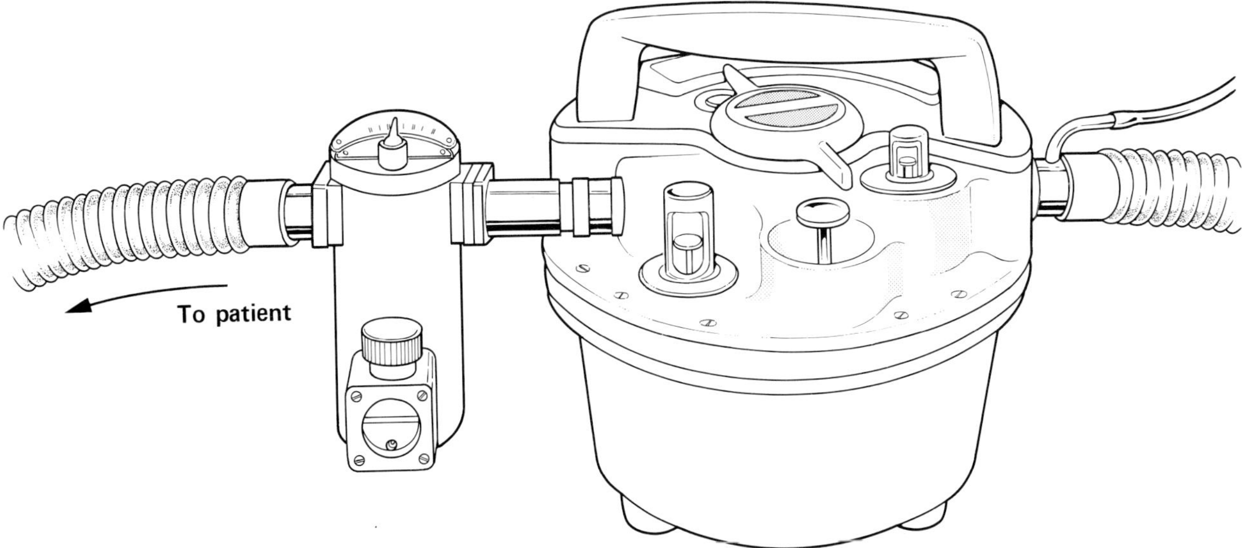

Fig. 7.5. The OMV connected to the outlet port of the EMO.

breathing system contains several valves: one valve connects the patient's airway to the system; another one or two are built into the SIB; and certain vaporizers, for example the Afya and PAC systems, have their own one-way valves.

In principle, at least two valves are needed in a breathing system to make gas flow in the correct direction. A universal breathing valve (see Fig. 2.9, page 24) at the patient's end of the system ensures that, during spontaneous or controlled ventilation, gas always reaches the patient from the vaporizer and passes out into the atmosphere (or to an antipollution system). You are strongly recommended to use a universal breathing valve for all patients. [Beware of confusing the Ambu E1 (anaesthesia) valve with the E2 (resuscitation only) valve (Fig. 7.6). The E2 valve is of no use for anaesthesia, as it allows the patient to breathe in atmospheric air from downstream. The anaesthetic valve has two sets of yellow valves inside, the resuscitation valve only one.]

A second one-way valve is needed to prevent gas from flowing into the vaporizer, rather than into the patient, during IPPV. In the Afya and PAC systems, this second valve is attached to or built into the vaporizer itself (see ⑥ in Fig. 7.3, page 61) and the SIB can be mounted on a T-piece. The EMO does not have built-in one-way valve and must therefore be connected in series with the SIB, which does have its own valve and can prevent gas flowing backwards to the vaporizer (Fig. 7.7).

The breathing tubes that form the system are connected to the vaporizers and SIB by conically tapered metal or plastic connectors (ISO 22 mm diameter, 1 degree taper). Connections should be made firmly without excessive force. Study the diagrams of breathing systems in Fig. 7.7. It will help you understand the function of the breathing valve if you draw your own diagram of it from the manufacturer's instructions. If you are unsure about the assembly of the system, try breathing through it yourself (with the vaporizers turned off!).

Self-inflating bags or bellows

Several of the different types of SIB available are shown in Fig. 2.8 on page 23. All SIBs have a one-way valve upstream of the bag or bellows; gases can enter the SIB through this valve, but must leave through the other end of the SIB in the direction of the patient. The Oxford inflating bellows also has a one-way valve located downstream from the bellows.

The Oxford inflating bellows should be placed in the breathing system between the vaporizer and the breathing valve. During storage, the bellows is held down by a light internal clip, which is released by pulling upwards on the knob on top of the bellows. An internal spring will then tend to keep the bellows at about a third of its maximum capacity. The patient is free to inspire through the bellows.

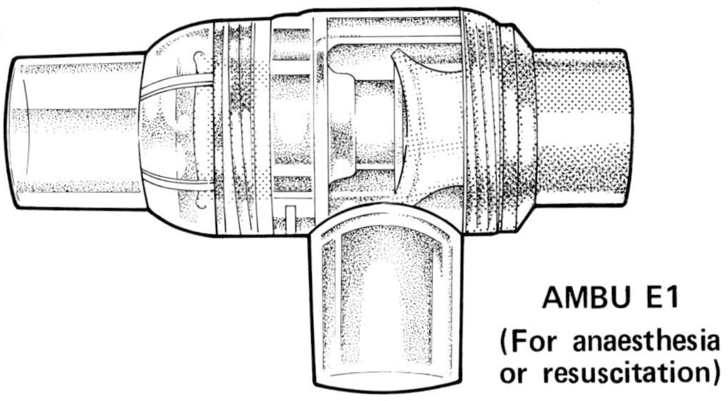

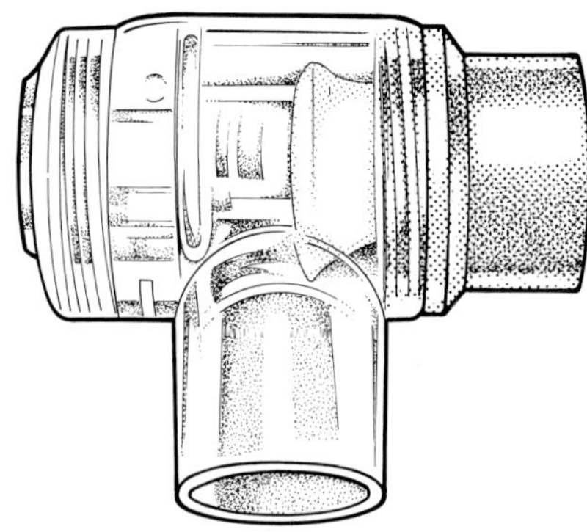

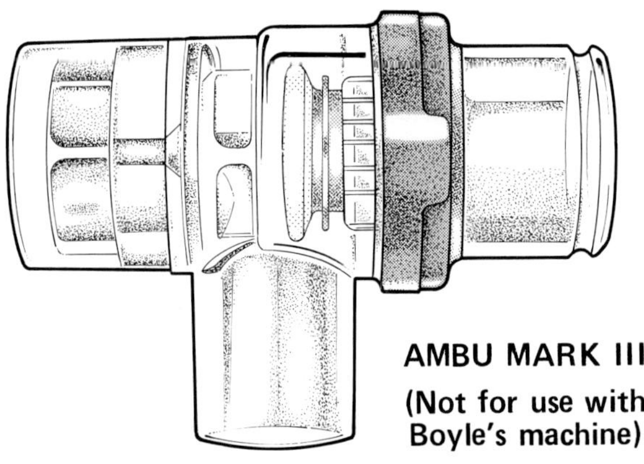

Fig. 7.6. Types of Ambu valve.

Because the system has a low resistance to flow, only a small movement of the bellows will be noticed, since air enters the bellows almost as fast as it leaves when the patient breathes in.

During controlled ventilation, lift the bellows slightly from the "rest" position and press down to inflate the patient's lungs. Inspiration should be started sharply to ensure that the breathing valve snaps smartly into the inspiratory position. Do not press down too hard at the end of inspiration, or the clip will engage and lock the bellows down. It is not necessary to lift the bellows to its maximum capacity, as this would produce a tidal volume of 2 litres, far in excess of the patient's need. At the base of the bellows is a small tap or nipple labelled "oxygen inlet", which was originally intended to allow the addition of oxygen during resuscitation. It is not compatible with modern universal breathing valves and should not be used (for the recommended technique of adding oxygen with an SIB, see Fig. 2.10, page 25). For paediatric use, a small-volume bellows is available that can be exchanged for the adult one on the same base and valves.

To allow a universal breathing valve to work properly with the Oxford inflating bellows, you must disable the one-way valve located downstream from the bellows, i.e., at the end of the bellows nearest the patient, by clipping the magnet supplied over the valve, thus lifting the valve disc to the top of the chamber. As a permanent alternative, the valve disc could be removed altogether. If you do not disable this valve, the breathing valve may stick and the patient will be harmed.

In some hospitals you may find that there are no universal breathing valves and that only a Heidbrink valve (also called an expiratory or pop-off valve) is available. This valve has no mechanism for preventing the patient's expired gas from flowing backwards to the SIB. It is not recommended for IPPV, but it can

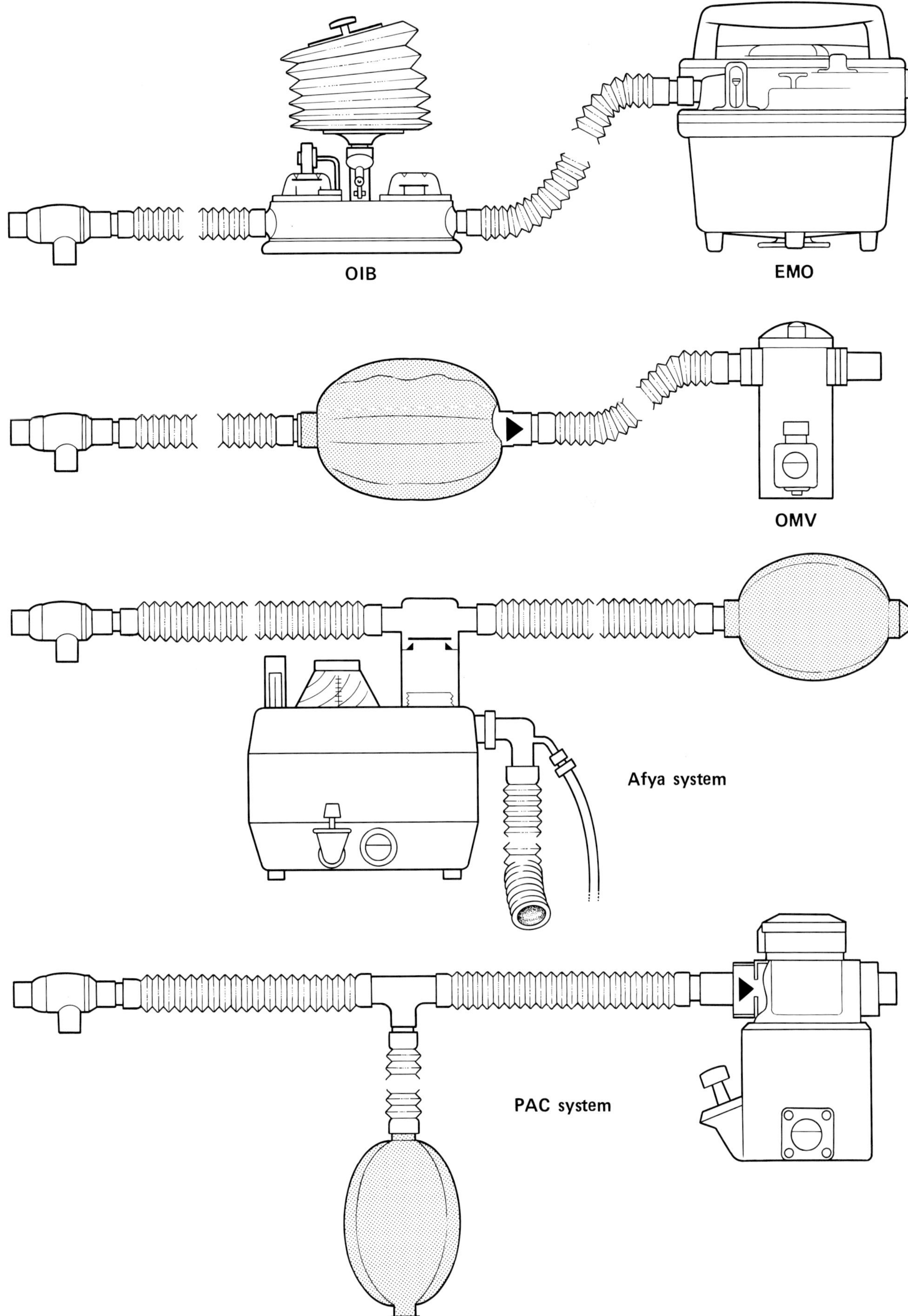

Fig. 7.7. Breathing systems (OIB, Oxford inflating bellows).

be used for spontaneous breathing with an Oxford inflating bellows (but not with any other SIB). In these circumstances, both the valves on the Oxford inflating bellows are needed, so remove the magnet from above the downstream valve and place it in the holder at the side. The valve is then free to move and will prevent the patient's expired gas from passing back into the bellows (Fig. 7.8).

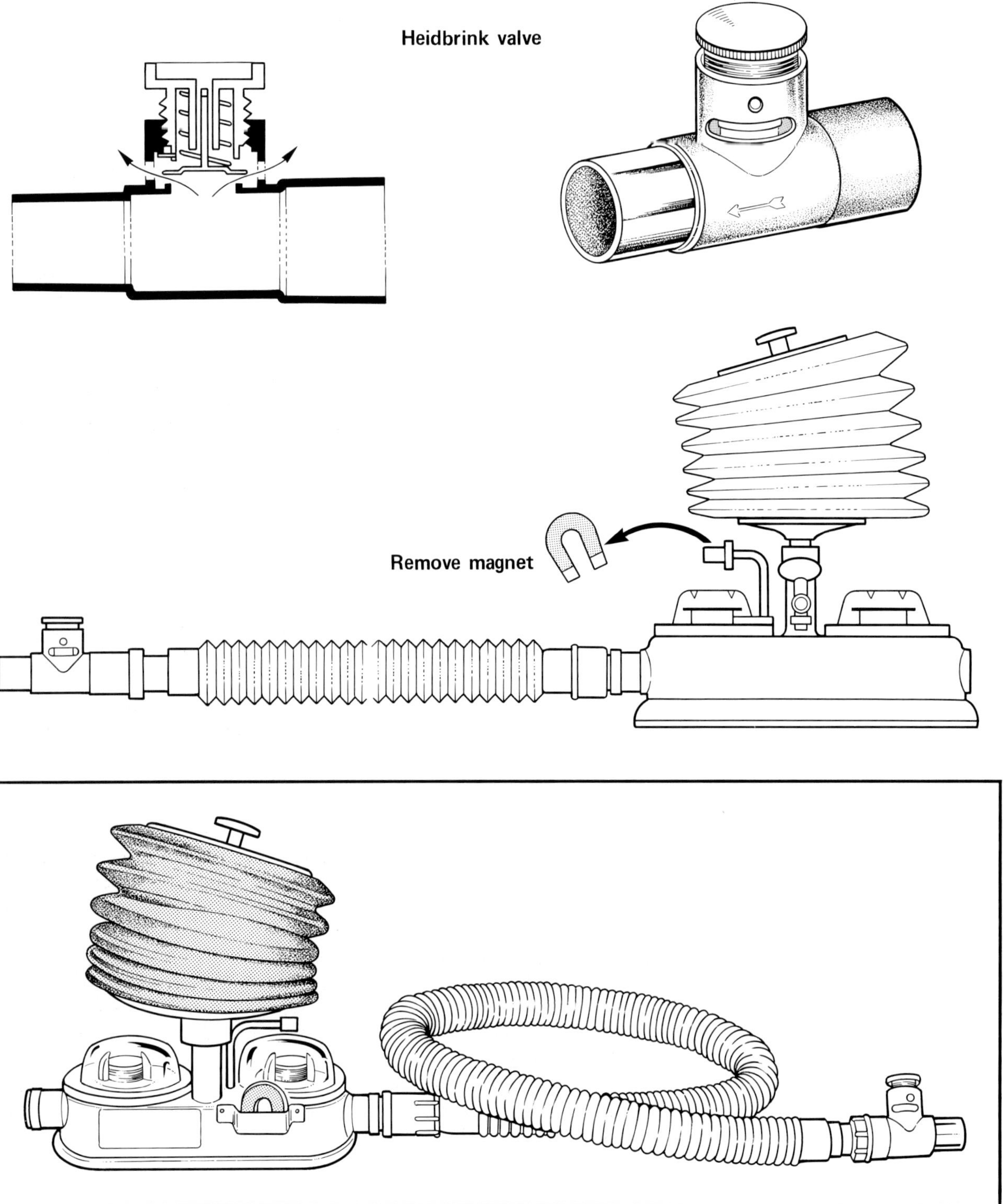

Fig. 7.8. Use of the Heidbrink valve with the Oxford inflating bellows after removal of the magnet.

Ambu, Cardiff, Laerdal, and similar bags can be used in a similar way to the Oxford inflating bellows. The bag is fitted with an inlet valve that allows gas or atmospheric air to enter at one end; for anaesthesia this valve is connected with a breathing tube to the vaporizer. This type of bag must always be used with a universal breathing valve, and never with a Heidbrink or a "resuscitation only" valve. Some bags have a port to allow direct connection of an oxygen supply, but, as with the Oxford inflating bellows, this is not recommended for oxygen enrichment; a T-piece and reservoir should be used instead.

With the Afya and PAC systems, a non-return valve is incorporated in the vaporizer itself and the SIB is mounted on a T-piece limb, which makes it easier to handle than an in-line bag (Fig. 7.7). A universal breathing valve must always be used for both spontaneous ventilation and IPPV.

Adding oxygen to the draw-over system

Air contains 20.9% oxygen and is perfectly adequate to oxygenate a healthy patient receiving draw-over anaesthesia, particularly if ether (which stimulates both respiration and cardiac output) is in use or if controlled ventilation is given with light general anaesthesia and a muscle relaxant.

If the patient is very young, old, or sick or if agents that cause cardiorespiratory depression, such as halothane, are given, then oxygen should always be added. Oxygen is usually available, even if only in limited quantities. Air (the carrier gas) already contains 20.9% oxygen, and oxygen enrichment is very economical in that the addition of only 1 litre/min can increase the oxygen concentration in the inspired gas to 35%–40%. With oxygen enrichment at 5 litres/min, a concentration of 80% can be achieved. Industrial-grade oxygen, for example as used for welding, is perfectly acceptable for the enrichment of a draw-over system and has been widely used for this purpose. (Industrial and medical oxygen are both prepared by the same process — the fractional distillation of air.)

To add oxygen to the breathing system, use a T-piece and reservoir tube at the vaporizer inlet (Fig. 7.9). If a ready-made T-piece with reservoir is unavailable, you can easily make an alternative using a small-bore oxygen tube threaded into a large-bore tube (Fig. 2.10B, page 25). Connect the T-piece and reservoir tube (or your improvised alternative) to the vaporizer inlet and turn on the oxygen supply. In this way the oxygen that flows from the cylinder during expiration is not wasted, but is stored in the reservoir tube for the next inspiration. The reservoir tubing should of course be open to the atmosphere at its free end to allow the entry of air, and it should be at least 30 cm long.

The Farman entrainer

This ingenious device uses the Venturi principle, by which an oxygen jet entrains room air in much larger quantities (1:10) to produce a flow of oxygen-enriched air. Connecting this device to the inlet of a draw-over system effectively converts the system to a continuous-flow mode, with the valves in the Oxford inflating bellows or similar SIB preventing retrograde flow. Use of the EMO system in continuous-flow mode is sometimes desirable in paediatric anaesthesia (see page 110). The entrainer is connected to an oxygen supply and the flow increased until a blood pressure gauge attached to the side-arm indicates a pressure (upstream) of 100 mmHg (13.3 kPa) (Fig. 7.10). A flow of 10 litres/min of oxygen-enriched air will then be produced — there is no need for a separate, flow-measuring apparatus — and the system can be used with an Ayre's T-piece for paediatric anaesthesia. If the Oxford inflating bellows is used in this mode, the magnet should be taken *off*.

Oxygen concentrators

The recent development of a zeolite molecular sieve capable of physically separating oxygen and nitrogen from air has made it possible to provide a relatively compact source of oxygen that is dependent only on a supply of mains electricity

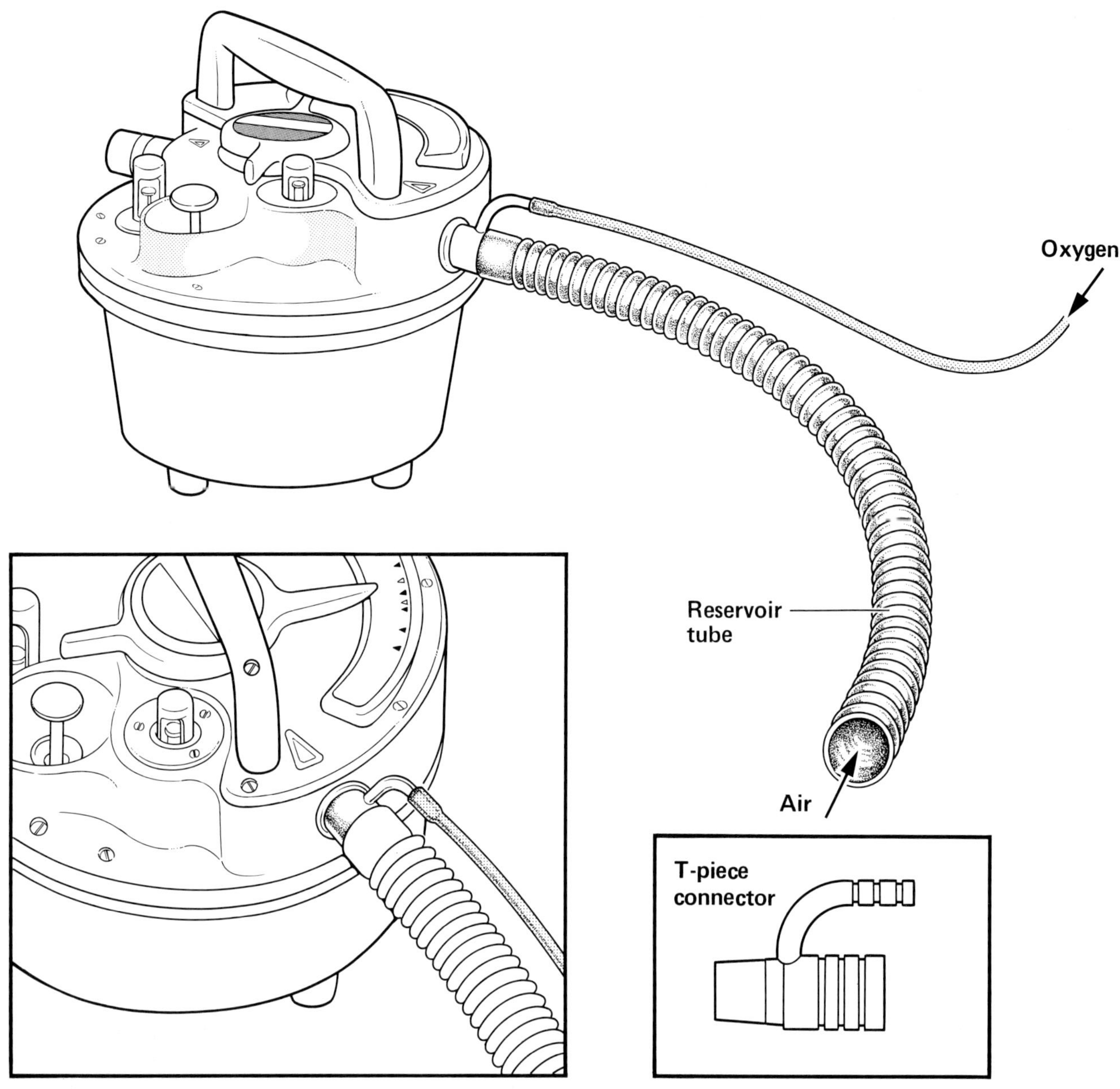

Fig. 7.9. Addition of oxygen with a T-piece and reservoir tube.

(Fig. 7.11; see also Fig. 15.1, page 127). There may be logistic problems in operating these units in small hospitals, such as difficulties with servicing or a humid climate, but they provide a potentially reliable supply of oxygen without the need for transporting cylinders over long distances at high cost. Further development of these devices is in progress. Another possibility for the future is a device that produces oxygen chemically by the catalytic splitting of hydrogen peroxide.

Standardization and identification of oxygen cylinders

An international standard exists for the identification of oxygen cylinders, which specifies that they should be painted white. Unfortunately, the standard is widely ignored. Medical oxygen cylinders originating in the United States of America are normally green, while those originating in Commonwealth countries are usually black with white shoulders. Cylinders of industrial oxygen should also be identified clearly, but this is not always the case. Never use any cylinder to supply gas to a patient unless you are sure of its contents.

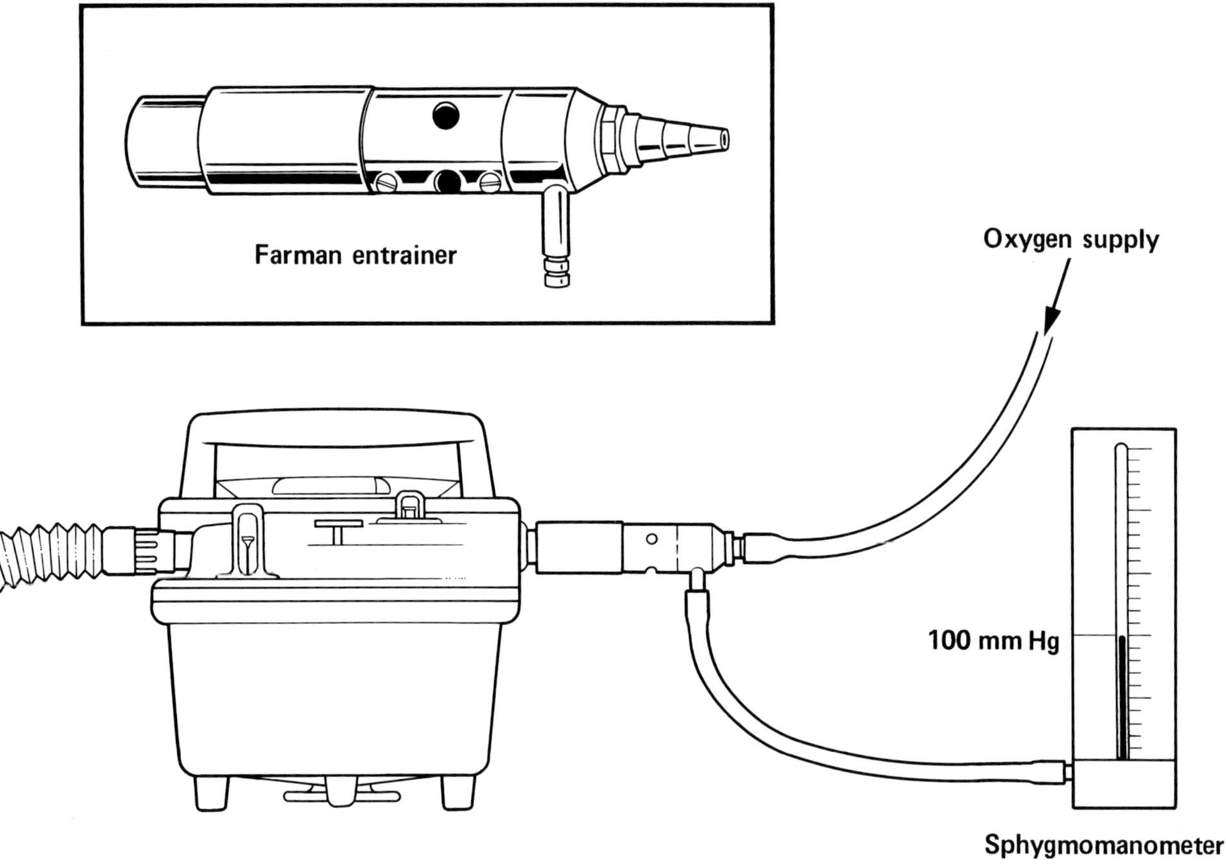

Fig. 7.10. Use of the Farman entrainer.

Oxygen, fire, and explosion risks

All operating theatre staff should be concerned about the possibility of fire or explosions in the operating theatre as a result of the use of anaesthetic vapours. It is important to distinguish between gas mixtures that are flammable, i.e., can burn, and those that are explosive. Explosions are much more dangerous to both staff and patients. Of the inhalational anaesthetics mentioned in this book, only one — ether — is flammable or explosive in clinical concentrations (though 10% trichloroethylene will burn in oxygen).

Mixtures of ether and air in the concentrations used for anaesthesia are flammable, but there is no concentration of ether that will explode when mixed only with air. However, if either oxygen or nitrous oxide is added to ether, the mixture becomes explosive.

There is no site within the draw-over apparatus itself where ether combustion could start. The point of risk is therefore the place where the patient's expired gas enters the room, before the ether is diluted by air. If you are using 3–5% ether as an anaesthetic in combination with a muscle relaxant, it is likely that the ether concentration in the patient's expired gas will be less than the lowest flammable concentration (2%). When flammable gases are in use, the most likely source of combustion in the operating theatre is the surgical diathermy machine and other electrical apparatus, followed by static electricity, which is unlikely to start a fire, but can trigger an explosion if the appropriate gas mixtures are present. No potential cause of combustion or source of sparking should be allowed within 30 cm of any expiratory valve through which a potentially flammable or explosive mixture is escaping. The use of diathermy outside this "zone of risk" is generally acceptable, but if explosive mixtures are in use, for example ether/oxygen or ether/nitrous oxide/oxygen, diathermy should be avoided. It should, of course, never be used inside the mouth or thorax if ether is in use.

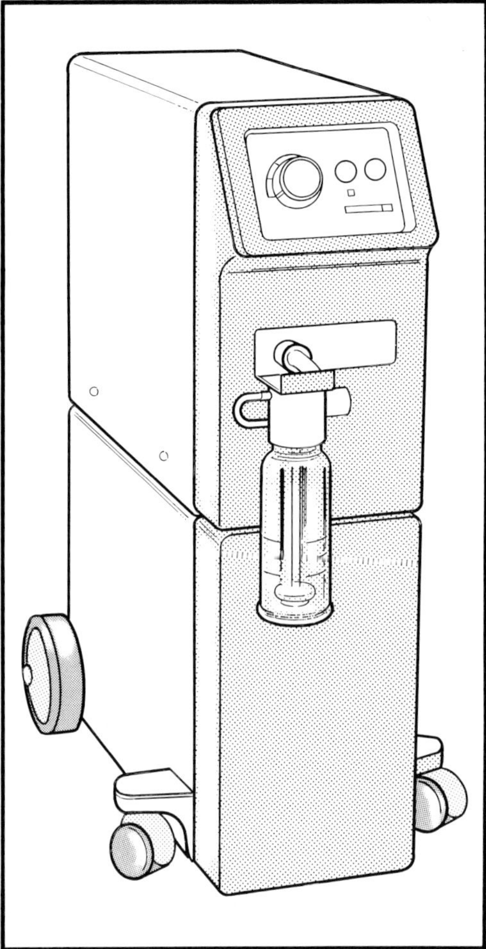

Fig. 7.11. Oxygen concentrator.

What reasonable precautions should you take?

If possible, your operating theatre and equipment should be of the antistatic type. This is important in a dry climate, but less so in a humid one where there is a natural antistatic coating of moisture.

Electrical sockets and switches should either be spark-proof or be situated at least 1 m above floor level.

The patient's expired gases should be carried away from the expiratory valve down wide-bore tubing at least to the floor (ether is heavier than air) or out of the operating theatre. Make sure that no one stands on the hose and that there is nothing that could trigger combustion near the end of this tubing. If you use oxygen enrichment during induction, but not surgery, the patient's expired gas will cease to be explosive within 3 min of stopping the addition of oxygen.

Continuous-flow machines

Continuous-flow anaesthetic machines (commonly known as Boyle's machines or simply gas machines) are in widespread use. They rely on a supply of compressed medical gas, either from cylinders attached directly to the machine or piped from a large bank of cylinders or liquid oxygen supply elsewhere in the hospital. The two gases most commonly used are oxygen and nitrous oxide. Cylinders are attached to the machine by a special yoke that prevents the connection of the nitrous oxide supply to the oxygen port and vice versa — the pin-index system. Some older machines may lack this system, and extreme care is needed in their use to prevent incorrect connections. The cylinders contain gas at high pressure, which is reduced to the anaesthetic machine's working pressure, usually 400 kPa (4 atmospheres), by a reducing valve. Each gas then passes through a needle valve at the base of a rotameter. This valve controls the flow of gas to the patient, once the cylinder valve has been opened with a key or spanner to allow gas to flow out. The gas passes through the rotameter, which measures the gas flow by upward displacement of a bobbin in a tube, and along the "back bar" at the top of the machine, where it may be diverted through a vaporizer for the addition of a volatile anaesthetic agent (Fig. 7.12). A separate switch or tap is usually provided to allow for a high flow of oxygen to be delivered to the patient in case of emergency, bypassing the rotameters and vaporizers. Gas is delivered from the common gas outlet at the top or front of the machine, to which a breathing system is connected.

The vaporizers on a Boyle's machine may be of the calibrated, thermocompensated type (for example Fluotec) or simple Boyle's bottles, which are usually used for ether (Fig. 7.13). The Boyle's bottle is uncalibrated, and its output declines as the ether becomes cold. It has two controls: a lever that diverts gas from the back bar down a tube into the vaporizer, and a hood that can be depressed to make the gases pass closer to or even bubble through the liquid ether. Always start with the hood up, increasing the concentration with the lever first, and then lowering the hood if necessary. Never bubble anaesthetic gas through any agent other than ether. Remember that with a Boyle's bottle the output is neither calibrated nor constant, so you will have to watch the patient with special care. Ether used in a Boyle's machine always produces a potentially explosive mixture.

The Magill breathing system

This system, which incorporates a Heidbrink valve, is in common use on continuous-flow machines (Fig. 7.14). It is suitable only for spontaneously breathing patients and requires a total gas flow from the rotameters that is approximately equal to the patient's minute volume, for example nitrous oxide at 4 litres/min and oxygen at 2 litres/min for an adult. Always give at least 30% oxygen to provide a margin of safety should there be any inaccuracy in the rotameters. If you wish to give IPPV with a Boyle's machine, you must use a different breathing system; the Magill system can be modified simply by exchanging the Heidbrink

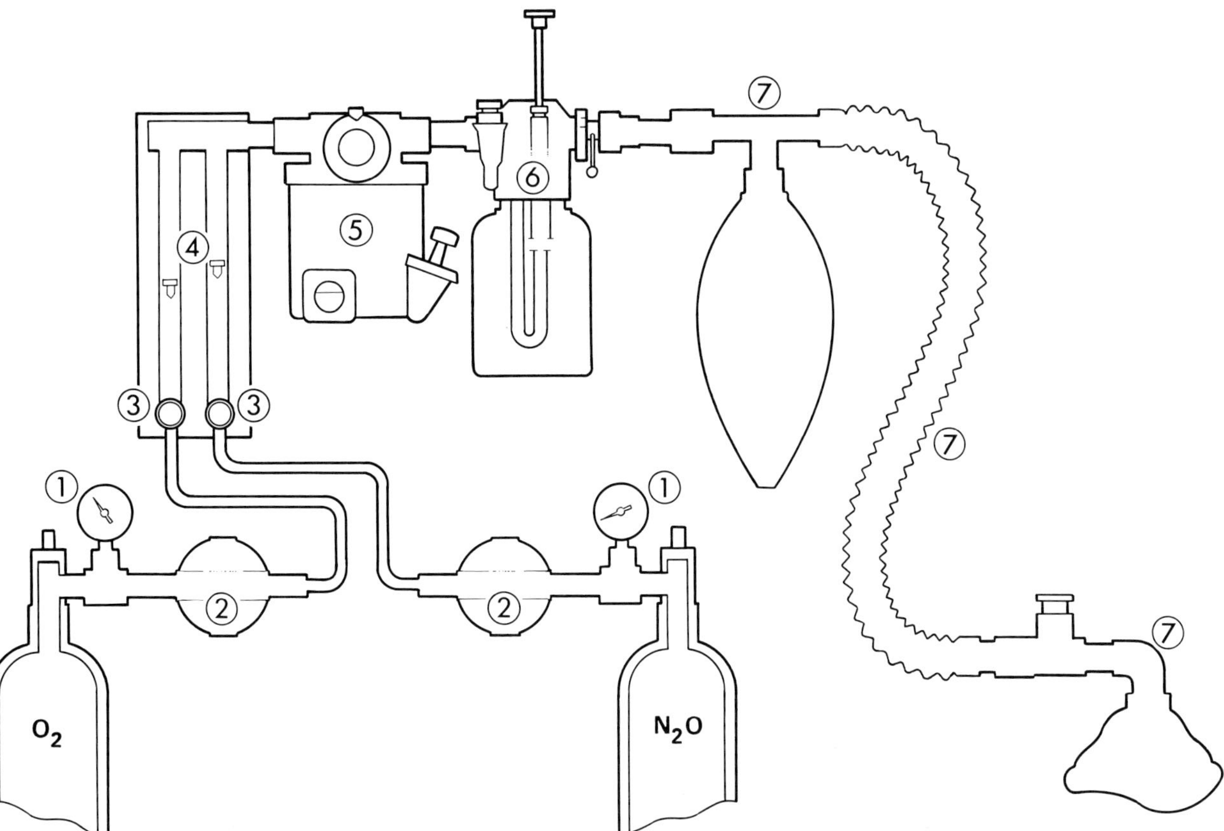

Fig. 7.12. Gas pathway on a continuous-flow (Boyle's) machine with a compressed gas supply. (1) Pressure gauges, (2) reducing valves, (3) flow-control (needle) valves, (4) rotameters, (5) calibrated vaporizer, (6) Boyle's bottle, (7) Magill breathing system.

valve for a suitable universal breathing valve such as an Ambu E1 or Ruben valve. Squeezing the reservoir bag will then inflate the patient's lungs. The patient can also take a spontaneous breath from the bag, so the modified system is suitable for both controlled and spontaneous respiration.

DANGER: Do *not* use a Laerdal IV, Ambu Mark III, or other similar valve with low switching-flow in this way, as it will jam on a continuous-flow system.

If you have to give IPPV with a Boyle's machine and a suitable universal breathing valve is not available, there are some other possible methods, though they are much less efficient and convenient.

1. If you are using a face mask, you can close the Heidbrink (expiratory) valve, squeeze the reservoir bag to inflate the lungs, and then lift the edge of the face mask to allow the patient to breathe out directly into the atmosphere. It takes skill to ventilate the lungs properly in this way.

2. If the patient is to be intubated, use an endotracheal connector with a suction port (such as a Cobb's connector). You can then inflate the lungs by squeezing the bag and occluding the open port with your finger; to allow expiration, remove your finger from the hole.

3. For brief periods only (less than 5 min), you can ventilate with a Magill system by screwing the Heidbrink valve about half closed and squeezing the bag to inflate the lungs. Gas escapes through the valve during both inspiration and expiration. This method is very inefficient in that a high flow of fresh gas of at least 10–15 litres/min is needed, which will soon exhaust your supplies. There is also considerable rebreathing of expired gas, which is bad for the patient.

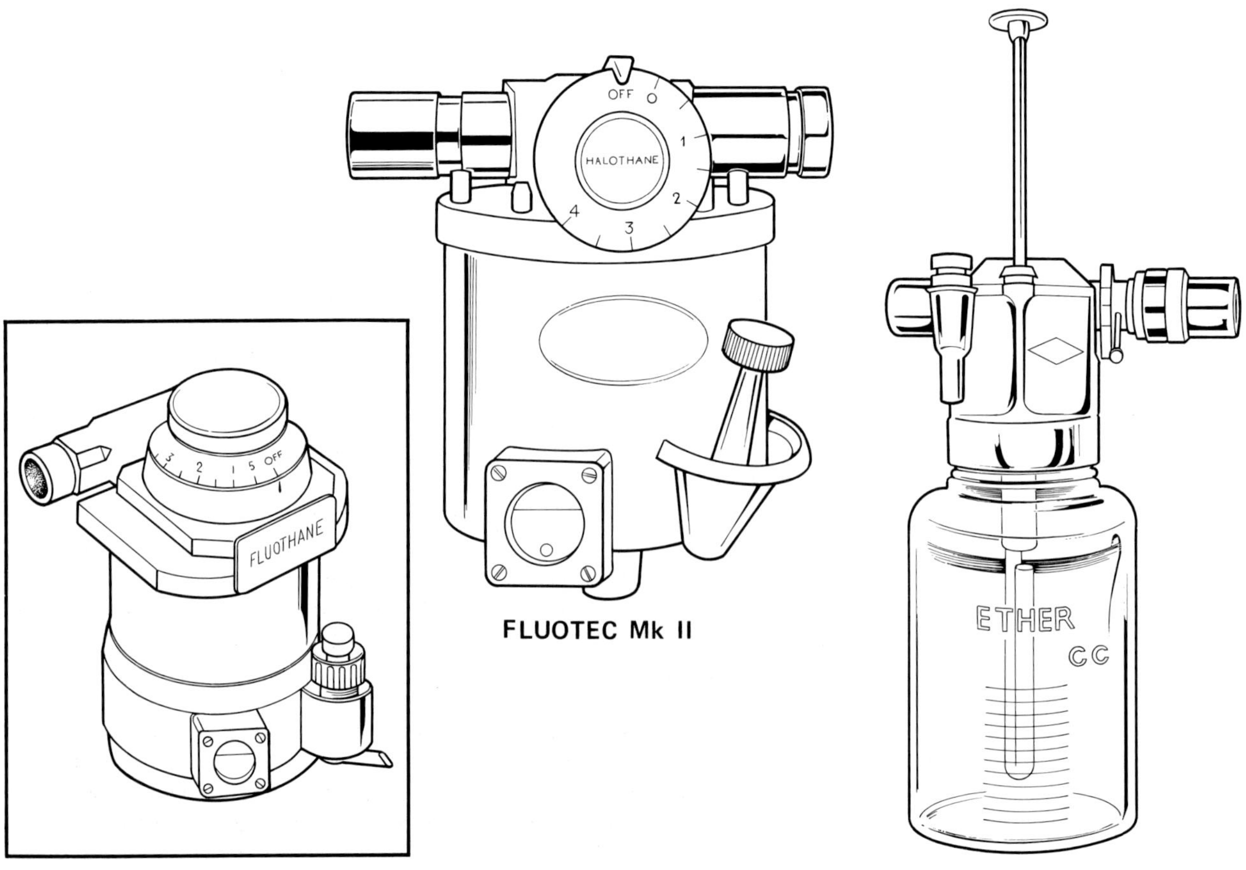

Fig. 7.13. **Some vaporizers used on continuous-flow machines with compressed gas supplies.**

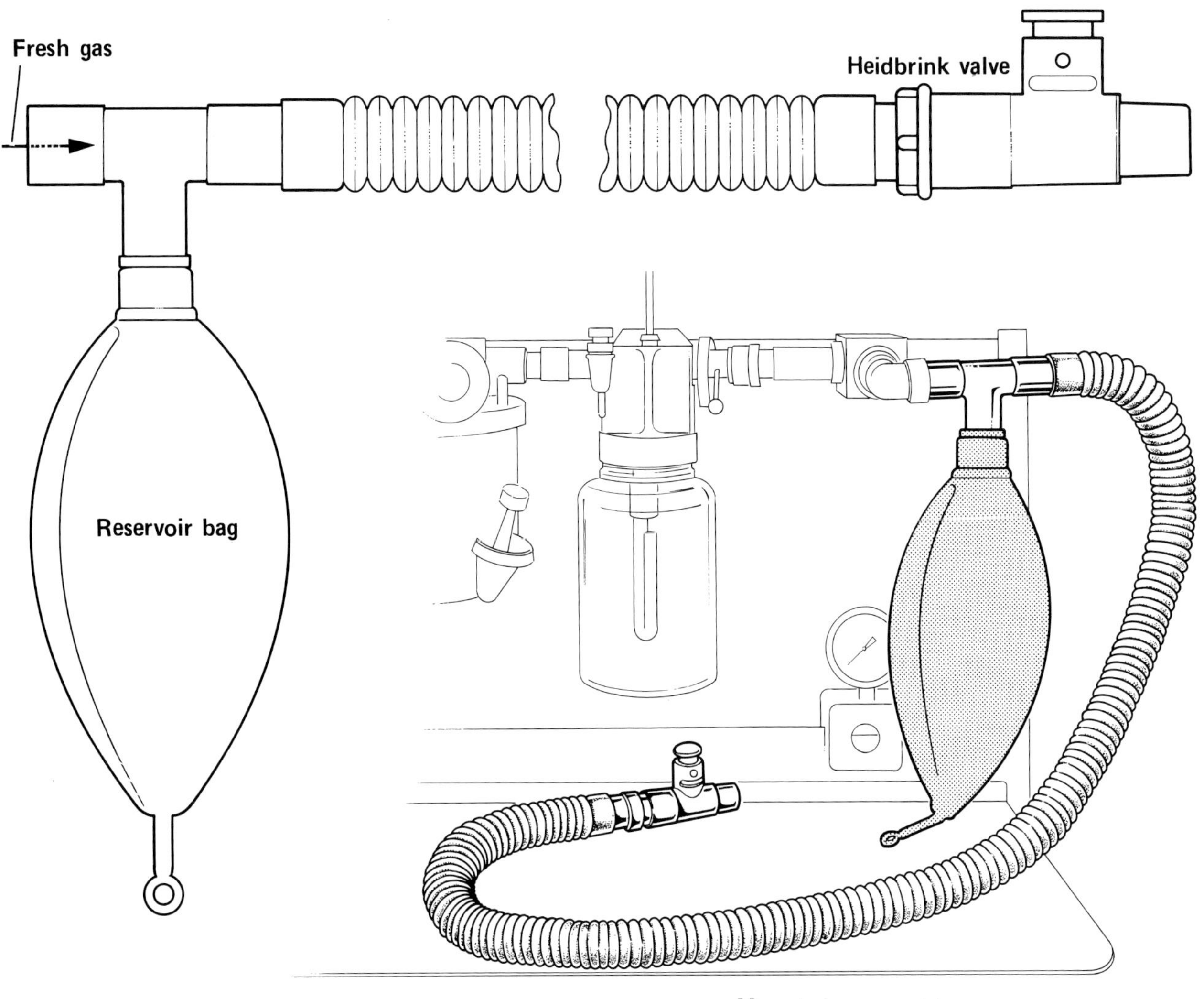

Fig. 7.14. Magill breathing system.

Checking your apparatus

Before beginning anaesthesia, you must thoroughly check the machine, with reference to the check-list in Annex 2 (a copy of which should be fixed permanently to your machine). Ensure that you have sufficient compressed gas for the operation, and at least one spare cylinder of oxygen. You must also have an SIB with which to ventilate the lungs should your machine fail. Also check other essential apparatus such as the laryngoscope and sucker. Then assemble the breathing system and test it for leaks by covering the end with your hand and squeezing the reservoir bag. No gas should escape if the Heidbrink valve is closed. (Remember to open it again afterwards!) At least once a month, check the whole machine and any gas hoses for leaks by "painting" suspect areas with soapy water and observing whether bubbles form when you turn on the gas supply. Continuous-flow machines are prone to leakage because the gases are kept at relatively high pressures inside them.

All types of apparatus should be kept in a clean and dust-free environment, away from extremes of temperature, and covered when not in use. Vaporizers should be drained of anaesthetic if they are unlikely to be used for a week or more. Put a cork or spigot in the end of any gas port or tubing during storage to prevent the entry of insects. Regular cleaning, inspection, and simple maintenance will familiarize you with your equipment, as well as help to keep it in good order. Try to estimate when new parts will be required, and order spares well in advance, before the machine breaks down and leaves you in difficulty.

8 Specimen general anaesthetic techniques

This chapter contains examples of general anaesthetic techniques that should be feasible in small or medium-sized hospitals. The descriptions are intended as guidelines, rather than as instructions to be followed in every detail. (For more information about the drugs recommended, see Chapter 9.)

General inhalational anaesthesia

With intubation, muscle relaxation, and artificial ventilation

This can be regarded as a *universal technique* that is suitable for any operation on an adult patient lasting more than 20 min, especially when rapid recovery is required. It is *contraindicated* when difficult intubation is anticipated. In such cases, use an inhalational induction/intubation technique (for example as described on pages 54–57), and then proceed from step 4.

1. Pre-oxygenate the patient by giving him or her a high concentration of oxygen to breathe for at least 3 min, or 10 breaths of pure oxygen at a flow of 10 litres/min from a closely fitting anaesthetic face mask. Loading the lungs with oxygen in this way allows the patient to remain well oxygenated even if endotracheal intubation takes several minutes.

2. Induce anaesthesia with a sleep dose of thiopental, usually 4–5 mg/kg of body weight for an adult, injected intravenously over 30–45 s.

3. Intubate the trachea after producing muscle relaxation with suxamethonium (1 mg/kg of body weight). Ventilate with 10% ether in air for 3 min to establish inhalational anaesthesia.

4. When the effect of suxamethonium wears off, usually after 3–5 min, give an appropriate dose of a "non-depolarizing" relaxant, such as alcuronium or gallamine.

5. Ventilate with 3% ether in air using a draw-over system and IPPV; surgical diathermy may be used. Halothane 1–1.5% or trichloroethylene 0.5–1% may be used in place of ether, in which case oxygen supplementation is strongly advised.

6. Five minutes before the end of surgery, turn off the ether supply and ventilate with air.

7. At the end of surgery, reverse the relaxant effects with 2.5 mg of neostigmine plus 1 mg of atropine given intravenously. Muscle relaxation cannot be reversed for 20 min after the relaxants have been given. You should normally wait until there is some evidence of returning muscle tone, such as slight respiratory movement, before giving neostigmine and atropine.

8. Continue to assist breathing until the patient breathes deeply and regularly and the mucous membranes are pink.

9. Turn the patient into the lateral position and extubate when he or she is awake, after careful suction of secretions from the mouth and pharynx.

With intubation and spontaneous breathing

This is an alternative technique for operations lasting less than an hour and not requiring relaxation.

1. Pre-oxygenate the patient as above.

2. Induce anaesthesia with a sleep dose of thiopental.

3. Intubate the patient after producing muscle relaxation with suxamethonium. If using ether, ventilate with 10% ether in air until breathing resumes, and then gradually decrease the ether concentration to 6%. The aim of this manoeuvre is to "load" the patient with ether while the suxamethonium is still acting, so that he or she will not cough and strain when breathing returns.

4. Allow the patient to breathe spontaneously *either* halothane 1% plus trichloroethylene 0.5% with oxygen enrichment at 1 litre/min *or* ether 6% in air.

5. At the end of surgery, extubate when the patient is *either* deeply anaesthetized (increase the anaesthetic concentration in the inspired gas to 10% ether or 3% halothane for 2 min before extubation) *or* awake. Always extubate with the patient in the lateral position after careful suction of secretions from the mouth and pharynx.

Without intubation

Intubation may not be necessary for patients requiring anaesthesia for a procedure lasting 10 min or less. Such patients must nevertheless be properly prepared and starved preoperatively. *Remember that there is no such thing as a "minor" anaesthetic.*

1. Place the patient in whichever lateral position gives best access to the operation site.

2. Induce anaesthesia with a sleep dose of thiopental.

3. Allow the patient to breathe halothane plus trichloroethylene in oxygen-enriched air from a face mask. Note that, if you have only ether available as an inhalational agent, it is much quicker to use an intubation technique, since it will take 15 min or more to settle the patient with ether given by face mask.

Ketamine anaesthesia

Ketamine given intravenously or intramuscularly as sole anaesthetic

This technique is suitable when muscle relaxation is not required, especially in children. It is also suitable as a "fall-back" technique if your inhalational apparatus (or gas supply for a Boyle's machine) fails or if you have to give a general anaesthetic without inhalational apparatus, for example at an accident for release of a trapped casualty.

1. Give a sedative drug and atropine as premedication (see page 50).

2. Insert an indwelling intravenous needle or cannula (in a struggling child it is more convenient to delay this until after ketamine has been given intramuscularly).

3. Give ketamine 8 mg/kg of body weight intramuscularly or 1–2 mg/kg intravenously (mixed with an appropriate dose of atropine, if not already given in premedication).

4. After intravenous injection of ketamine the patient will be ready for surgery in 1–2 min, and after intramuscular injection in 3–5 min.

5. Give incremental doses of ketamine if the patient responds to painful stimuli. Use half the original intravenous dose or a quarter of the original intramuscular dose.

6. At the end of the procedure, turn the patient into the lateral position for supervised recovery in a quiet place.

Ketamine infusion as part of a balanced anaesthetic technique with muscle relaxation

1. After premedication with atropine and pre-oxygenation, induce anaesthesia with a fast-running ketamine infusion containing 1 mg/ml (average adult dose 50–100 ml).

2. Give suxamethonium and intubate the trachea.

3. After breathing returns maintain anaesthesia with ketamine 1–2 mg/min (more if the patient has not received premedication) and give a non-depolarizing relaxant. Ventilate with air, enriched with oxygen if available.

4. At the end of surgery, reverse the muscle relaxation and extubate with the patient awake, as after inhalational anaesthesia.

General anaesthesia for emergency cases

The patient who requires anaesthesia for an emergency operation presents extra difficulties to the anaesthetist, who must make a full preoperative assessment and anticipate any likely problems. The patient may not have been fully prepared or be in an ideal physiological state. Certain pathological states, such as fluid depletion, can and must be rapidly treated before anaesthesia, but others, such as a chest infection, can be treated only within the limits of the time available, as excess delay would cause further deterioration of the patient's condition. Sick patients with poor circulation should receive smaller doses of almost every drug. (Suxamethonium is an exception; use a normal dose.) Be particularly careful with drugs given intravenously and local anaesthetics. Very often, the sicker the patient, the greater the risk associated with using spinal anaesthesia, so general anaesthesia may be preferable.

Patients requiring emergency surgery frequently have a full stomach. In an injured patient, gastric emptying will have stopped at the time of the injury. Patients with intra-abdominal disease and pregnant patients at or near term must also be assumed to have retained gastric contents with a high concentration of hydrochloric acid. If gastric contents enter the lungs during anaesthesia, severe damage and even death are real possibilities. One of your chief concerns must be to prevent this catastrophe. The presence in the trachea of a cuffed endotracheal tube is the only sure protection during general anaesthesia. This is one reason that so much stress is laid on endotracheal intubation in this book. The anaesthetist's goal is to insert the tube as swiftly and smoothly as possible, while keeping the lungs protected from both active vomiting and passive regurgitation.

The simplest way to intubate is with the patient awake, and this is almost always possible with neonates and infants aged less than 2 months, in whom it is the technique of choice. Many adults, especially if they are sick, will also tolerate intubation while awake if you explain what you intend to do and why. Use a well-lubricated laryngoscope blade, and insert it gently and slowly. When you can see the larynx (it may take a minute or two) pass the endotracheal tube through it, trying not to touch the sides of the pharynx on the way down, as this may make the patient gag and you will have to start again. On intubation the patient will probably cough, and your assistant may need to restrain the patient's hands. Immediately after intubation, you can safely induce anaesthesia with thiopental. (For an infant, you need only turn on the supply of inhalational anaesthetic agent.)

Rapid induction sequence

For emergency surgery, many anaesthetists prefer to use a "rapid induction sequence", sometimes called a "crash induction". The aim is to induce anaesthesia and intubate the trachea quickly and smoothly, while preventing regurgitation by external compression of the upper oesophagus.

First aspirate the stomach contents with a large gastric tube; this helps decompress the stomach, but does not guarantee to empty it. Remove the tube before proceeding, as it makes the gastro-oesophageal sphincter leak. Pre-oxygenate the patient, and check that an efficient suction apparatus is within reach and turned on (put the end of the sucker under the pillow). Your assistant should now press firmly backwards with finger and thumb on the patient's cricoid cartilage (Fig. 8.1). This cartilage forms a complete ring around the trachea in front of the upper oesophagus, and will thus compress and occlude the oesophagus, making regurgitation of gastric contents into the pharynx unlikely. Cricoid pressure must be maintained until you have intubated the patient, inflated the cuff, and tested it for leaks. *Make sure that your assistant understands this.* Once cricoid pressure has been applied, give the patient a previously calculated dose of thiopental by injecting it into the intravenous infusion tube, followed immediately by suxamethonium at 1 mg/kg of body weight. As soon as the patient relaxes, insert the laryngoscope and endotracheal tube; inflate the cuff, test it for leaks, and tie the tube into position.

A cuffed tube is not used in children aged less than 10 years, since the narrowest part of their airway is at the level of the cricoid cartilage, and a tube of the correct size will almost certainly fit this without the need for a cuff. If there is an air leak, pack the pharynx with moist ribbon gauze under direct vision using Magill's forceps. In children, it is especially important not to force in a tube that is too large, since the result will be oedema of the larynx after extubation. If a small leak of air round the tube during gentle inflation of the lungs can be heard, it is clear that the tube is not too tight. If, after intubation, you think that a smaller tube should have been used, change the tube immediately for a smaller one and little harm will have been done.

Even a cuffed tube cannot give absolute protection to the airway, so suck out any secretions from the mouth and pharynx before and after intubation and extubation.

Once you have successfully intubated the patient, you can proceed to any one of the possible anaesthetic plans outlined in Fig. 11.1, page 104. It is wise to reinsert the gastric tube and aspirate the stomach contents again. If the surgeon is operating in the abdomen, he or she can confirm that the tube has entered the stomach and can gently assist gastric emptying. Remember that at the end of the operation you must protect the patient's lungs by extubating with the patient awake and in the lateral position.

The rapid induction sequence described above is an important one with which both you and your assistant should be thoroughly familiar. It is harmless and not unpleasant for the patient, so you should practise it whenever possible on healthy patients for non-emergency operations to perfect your technique.

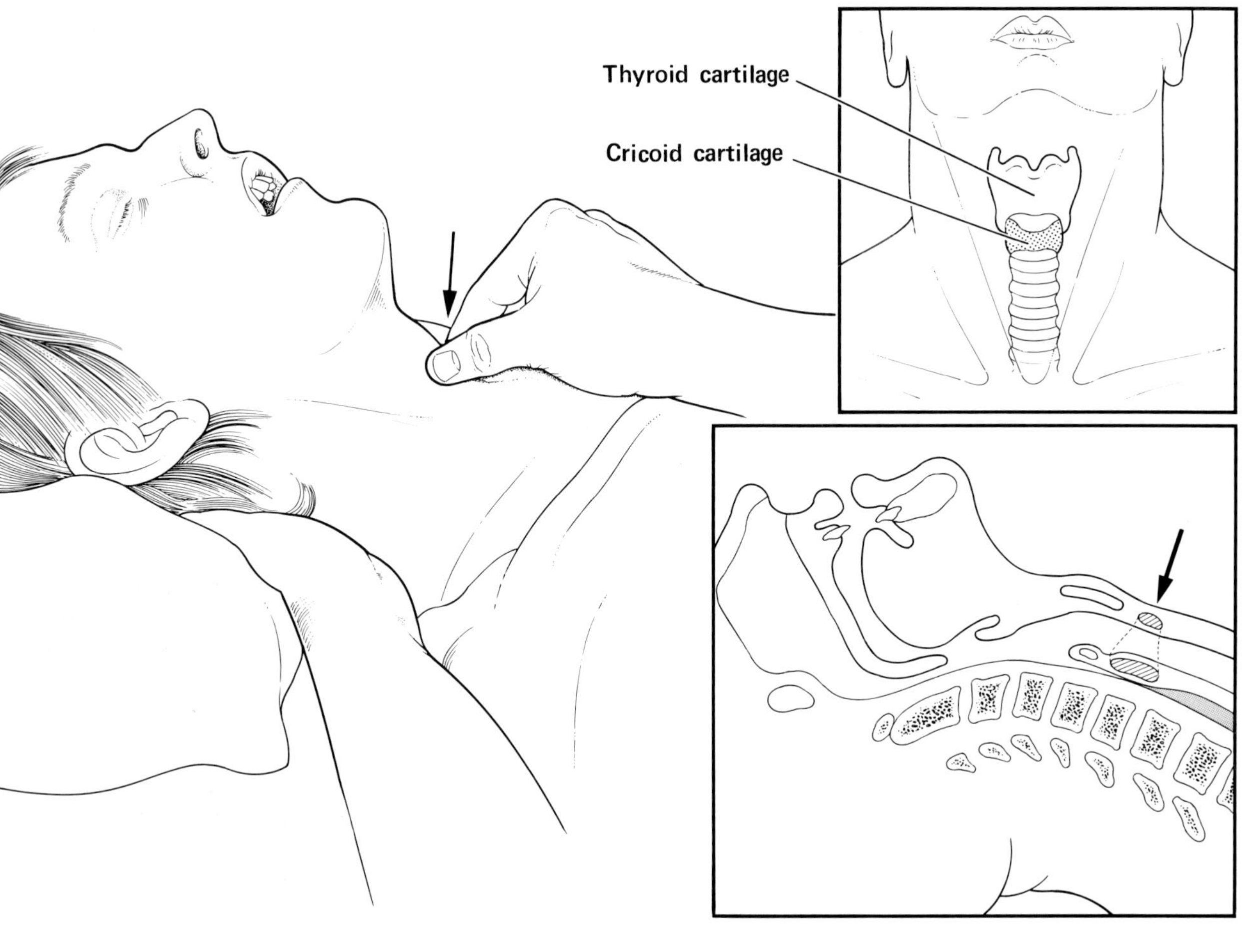

Fig. 8.1. Applying cricoid pressure to prevent regurgitation.

9 Drugs used in general anaesthesia

Inhalational agents

Diethyl ether ($CH_3.CH_2.0.CH_2.CH_3$)

Diethyl ether, commonly known simply as ether, is probably the most widely used inhalational agent in the world, because of its reputation (largely deserved) for safety, ready availability, and relatively low price. It is a colourless liquid with a strong, irritant smell and a boiling point of 35 °C. The concentrations used in anaesthesia vary from 2 to 20%. Ether is relatively soluble in blood, so the blood becomes saturated with the anaesthetic rather slowly; inhalational induction with ether is correspondingly slow, unless an additional agent such as halothane is used. Ether in anaesthetic concentrations is flammable when mixed with air and explosive when mixed with oxygen or nitrous oxide or both (see page 69). It should be stored in a cool, dark place.

Pharmacology

Ether has both anaesthetic and analgesic properties; the low concentrations that persist in the body after anaesthesia provide some relief from postoperative discomfort. During ether anaesthesia, there is an increase in catecholamine release from the adrenal glands, with an associated increase in cardiac output (except in very deep ether anaesthesia, when direct depression of the heart becomes more significant). Ether is safe to use when the surgeon wishes to infiltrate epinephrine or another vasoconstrictor drug. It produces muscle relaxation by an action similar to that of the non-depolarizing neuromuscular blocking drugs, whose effects it potentiates. It can be used as sole agent to produce sufficient muscular relaxation for laparotomy, though this requires deep anaesthesia, which results in slow postoperative recovery. Ether also produces some uterine relaxation in deep anaesthesia and may be used for external and internal version procedures in obstetrics. It is a bronchodilator and has been used to treat asthmatic attacks. When ether is given with a face mask, there is a marked increase in salivary secretion, which can be prevented by premedication with atropine. If secretions are profuse and are swallowed early in anaesthesia, the ether that has dissolved in them may cause gastric irritation and postoperative vomiting. There is certainly a higher incidence of postoperative nausea and vomiting after deep ether anaesthesia than after anaesthesia with other agents, but this is not the case after anaesthesia with a combination of 3% ether, a muscle relaxant, and IPPV, as described on page 74. Most (80–90%) of the ether that enters the body is exhaled again, the remainder being metabolized.

Anaesthesia with ether alone (including ether induction) produces the "classical" stages of anaesthesia:

Stage I — analgesia.

Stage II — confusion, dilated pupils, struggling, and the possibility of breath-holding and vomiting.

Stage III — surgical anaesthesia divided into planes 1–4 with a progressive increase in pupillary size; relaxation increases, starting with the abdominal and lower intercostal muscles and progressing upwards.

Stage IV — minimal diaphragmatic activity; blood pressure begins to fall; finally respiratory and cardiac arrest occurs.

It is rare to use ether unsupplemented in this way, because of the slow induction and recovery phases.

Halothane ($CF_3.CHClBr$)

Halothane is a halogenated hydrocarbon with a sweetish, non-irritant smell, which boils at 50 °C. The concentrations used in anaesthesia vary from 0.2 to 3%. It is a potent agent, and a calibrated vaporizer is necessary to avoid overdosage. Because it is less soluble in blood than ether, the blood becomes saturated more rapidly, so inhalational induction is relatively rapid and pleasant for the patient. If your supplies are limited, it is best to reserve halothane for facilitating inhalational induction or for settling a patient after intravenous induction, while you start giving ether. Halothane is neither flammable nor explosive in clinical conditions.

Pharmacology

Halothane produces a smooth induction of anaesthesia, but poor analgesia. Attempting to use it as sole agent for surgical anaesthesia is likely to result in severe cardiorespiratory depression with marked cyanosis, unless the inspired gas contains a high concentration of oxygen. Halothane can produce some muscular relaxation, though less than ether. Like ether, it relaxes the gravid uterus and is a bronchodilator. Depression of the respiratory centre by halothane usually produces shallow breathing at an increased rate; this increase in rate is less marked after opiate premedication. The main effect on the cardiovascular system is direct depression of the myocardium with a fall in cardiac output and blood pressure. However, there is marked skin vasodilatation, so the patient's tissues may appear well perfused. In a spontaneously breathing patient, the depressant effects on the heart are less marked than in a patient whose respiration is being assisted; in the former, retention of carbon dioxide (from respiratory depression) results in an increased secretion of catecholamines, whose cardiovascular effects tend to oppose the fall in cardiac output. Unfortunately, halothane also sensitizes the heart to the dysrhythmic effects of catecholamines, so dysrhythmias may occur. Surgical infiltration with epinephrine during halothane anaesthesia should therefore not be permitted.

Many of the disadvantages of halothane can be overcome by giving it in combination with an effective inhalational analgesic, such as nitrous oxide (50–70%) or trichloroethylene (0.5–1%).

Trichloroethylene ($CHCl.CCl_2$)

Trichloroethylene is a halogenated hydrocarbon with a sweet smell, which boils at 87 °C. In its anaesthetic formulation it is coloured with a blue dye.

Pharmacology

Trichloroethylene has potent analgesic properties, but when used alone it produces unconsciousness rather slowly because of a poor hypnotic effect and high blood solubility. It can be used, like halothane, to "smooth out" inhalational induction before the introduction of ether. If used as the sole anaesthetic agent without controlled ventilation, it produces cardiorespiratory depression with a tachypnoea. In analgesic doses it can be extremely useful; it has long been used for inhalational pain relief during labour, in concentrations of 0.35–0.5%. Analgesia with trichloroethylene in air can be useful for short, surface procedures, for example incising an abscess or changing a dressing for an outpatient. For more major procedures, 1% trichloroethylene can be used with muscle relaxants and IPPV with air or oxygen/air, as described on page 74. Like halothane, trichloroethylene is incompatible with infiltration of epinephrine.

Since trichloroethylene is a good analgesic, it can usefully be combined with halothane, which is a good hypnotic but has poor analgesic properties. Two suitable vaporizers (see page 55) can be connected in series with the trichloroethylene vaporizer nearer to the patient (Fig. 9.1); this system can provide excellent anaesthesia for spontaneously breathing patients with concentrations of halothane around 1% and trichloroethylene 0.5% (see page 75).

Methoxyflurane, enflurane, and isoflurane

These halogenated ethers have been introduced over the last 20 years in some parts of the world, but in view of their high cost and marginal advantages they are not recommended for use in small hospitals or rural areas. Like halothane, they are potent agents and should be given only from calibrated, agent-specific vaporizers.

Chloroform and ethyl chloride

Although these agents may still be available and in use in some parts of the world, they are extremely hazardous, particularly for the inexperienced anaesthetist, and their use cannot be recommended.

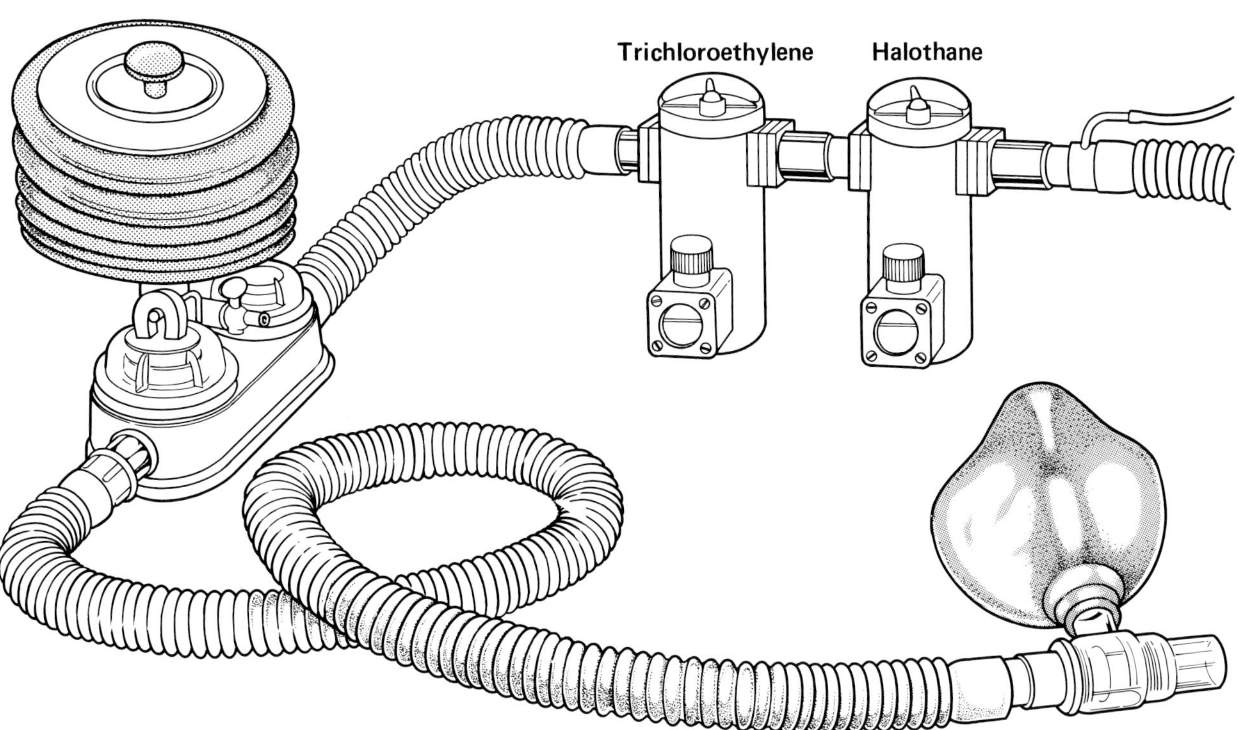

Fig. 9.1. Use of two vaporizers to combine the advantages of halothane and trichloroethylene.

Intravenous anaesthetics

Thiopental (thiopentone)

Thiopental is a thiobarbiturate, i.e., a sulfur-containing barbiturate, presented as a yellow powder and used as a 2.5% aqueous solution for inducing anaesthesia. The solution is strongly alkaline and irritant, and hence problems may arise if it is injected outside the vein. Like all barbiturates, thiopental depresses cerebral function, producing unconsciousness together with depression of the respiratory and vasomotor centres. The respiratory and vasomotor depression is relatively transient and mild in healthy patients given a sleep dose, but an overdose can cause hypotension or respiratory arrest. After a normal induction dose, anaesthesia is produced in one arm–brain circulation time — usually 15–25 s, but longer in elderly or hypovolaemic patients. Typically, the patient takes a deep breath or sighs just before losing consciousness. If a single dose is given, the patient will remain unconscious for about 4–7 min, but may react to painful stimulation towards the end of this time.

Recovery occurs because the drug passes out of the brain, where it is initially concentrated, into other tissues. Although barbiturates are eventually broken down in the liver, this takes several hours. Consequently, if repeated doses of thiopental are given, there will come a point where all the body's stores have become saturated, and the patient may then take many hours or even days to recover consciousness. Repeated doses of thiopental should therefore not be given to prolong anaesthesia. For a short procedure lasting only a minute or two, it is possible to use a single dose of thiopental as the sole anaesthetic, but beware of laryngeal spasm if the procedure is painful or causes vagal stimulation, for example anal dilatation.

Methohexital (methohexitone)

Methohexital is sometimes available as an alternative to thiopental. It is more potent, the powder being diluted to make a 1% solution, with an average sleep dose of 1 mg/kg of body weight. After a single dose, patients wake up more quickly than after thiopental, but there is still an element of "barbiturate hangover", and no patient who has been given either drug should drive a vehicle, operate machinery, or drink alcohol during the following 24 hours.

Ketamine

Ketamine is a unique drug. In anaesthetic doses, it produces a trance-like state of "dissociative anaesthesia", which consists of profound analgesia with only slightly impaired pharyngeal and laryngeal reflexes. There is sympathetic activation, with mild cardiovascular stimulation and small increases in arterial blood pressure, and also increases in intracranial and intraocular pressures. Like ether, ketamine is a bronchodilator, and when given in large doses by the intramuscular route, it produces profuse salivation, so atropine is usually given before or with it. It is oxytocic and should therefore not be given during pregnancy, except at term for forceps delivery or caesarean section. It does not provide any muscular relaxation; indeed the patient's limbs sometimes become fixed in abnormal positions because of altered muscle tone. The induction dose generally recommended is 1–2 mg/kg of body weight given intravenously (depending on premedication) or 6–8 mg/kg given intramuscularly. Several formulations of different strengths are available, but it is recommended that the 50 mg/ml strength be used as the standard, and diluted if required for intravenous use. The formulation of this strength is presented as a multidose ampoule, which should be refrigerated after opening.

For procedures requiring relaxation and also for more general use, ketamine can be given by infusion in conjunction with a muscle relaxant and IPPV with air. Ketamine provides light surgical anaesthesia in much the same way as 3% ether. Infusing the drug reduces the total dose needed and allows more rapid recovery. The average infusion rate used for an adult is about 1 mg/min.

In subanaesthetic doses of around 0.5 mg/kg of body weight, ketamine is an excellent analgesic and produces no clinical evidence of respiratory depression. It is particularly valuable for providing analgesia when it is necessary to move a patient with a painful lesion, for example to position a patient for conduction anaesthesia or to change a plaster or dressing. Ketamine has also found a special place as an anaesthetic for children in whom repeated anaesthesia is needed over a short period and when access to the airway may be difficult. No anaesthetic can guarantee a safe airway, but the airway is certainly less at risk during ketamine anaesthesia than with any other general anaesthetic technique. In a patient with a family history of malignant hyperthermia, ketamine may be safely used.

Ketamine's main drawbacks are its relatively high cost and limited availability. Hallucinations during recovery may be a problem (though rarely so in children), but do not occur if ketamine is used as induction agent only and is followed by a conventional inhalational anaesthetic. The incidence of hallucinations after ketamine is given as the sole anaesthetic agent can be reduced by suitable sedative premedication with a benzodiazepine or butyrophenone drug.

Opiate drugs

Opiate analgesics such as morphine (natural) and pethidine (synthetic) are frequently used in premedication. They are also of value in preventing reflex responses to painful stimulation during anaesthesia (shown in the paralysed patient by tachycardia, sweating, or a rise in blood pressure), particularly when light general anaesthesia with nitrous oxide is being used. (Analgesic supplements are rarely needed during ether anaesthesia.) As a supplement to anaesthesia, give small doses of opiate drugs intravenously (for example morphine 0.1 mg/kg or pethidine 0.25 mg/kg of body weight). Do not give increments of opiate in the last half-hour of surgery or you may have trouble getting the patient to start breathing again. Opiates depress respiration, usually by reducing the respiratory rate, with little effect on the depth of respiration. In the postoperative period, it is advisable to give at least the first dose of opiate analgesic intravenously, as the patient's responses, in terms of both analgesia and possible respiratory depression, can be closely watched and the dosage adjusted to the patient's needs more easily than if the drug is given intramuscularly.

Severely injured patients who require opiate analgesics should receive them only by the intravenous route, since absorption from other sites may be delayed because of poor perfusion. For example, an opiate drug injected intramuscularly may not produce adequate analgesia and a further dose may be given; when the circulation is restored and hence the perfusion of the injection site improved, all the drug will be absorbed at once, which may cause a collapse from opiate overdose.

Opiate overdose and antagonists

If an overdose of opiate is accidentally given, the main problem is likely to be respiratory depression. Primary treatment must always consist of artificial ventilation if necessary, using whatever apparatus is available. Naloxone is a specific opiate antagonist that can be given intravenously or intramuscularly and is capable of completely reversing the depressant effects of opiates. Its effects are briefer than those of morphine, particularly if it is given intravenously, and supplementary doses, preferably intramuscular, are recommended to prevent the return of the effects of morphine. Nalorphine is a cheaper alternative to naloxone, but it can produce respiratory depression in its own right if an overdose is given, so more care is needed.

Muscle relaxant drugs

These are drugs that act at the neuromuscular junction, blocking transmission of nerve impulses and causing muscular relaxation and paralysis. They have no effect on consciousness or sensation, so you must *never* give them to a conscious patient, nor to any other patient unless you are sure that you can ventilate the lungs with a face mask and also pass an endotracheal tube. Muscle relaxation during anaesthesia is required:

- to allow laryngoscopy and intubation during light anaesthesia
- to improve the surgeon's access to specific organs and tissues.

Physiology of neuromuscular transmission

When a motor nerve is stimulated, a wave of electrical depolarization passes along it as far as the nerve ending on the muscle (the motor end-plate). At this point the arrival of the electrical impulse triggers the release of a stored chemical transmitter, acetylcholine, which diffuses across the synaptic cleft and interacts with the muscle receptors, producing electrical depolarization, which leads to mechanical contraction of the muscle fibre. The acetylcholine is then broken down by an enzyme (acetylcholinesterase) or taken up again by the nerve ending.

Muscle relaxants resemble molecules of acetylcholine closely enough to bind to its receptors, but their effect after binding differs from that of acetylcholine.

Suxamethonium (succinylcholine)

Suxamethonium actually consists of two acetylcholine molecules joined together. It causes depolarization of the muscle fibres, which can be seen as a fine twitching (fasciculation) of all the muscles after an intravenous dose of 1 mg/kg of body weight, followed by profound relaxation, usually within 45 s of injecting the drug. After this initial action, the motor end-plates remain depolarized and the muscles therefore paralysed until the suxamethonium is broken down by the enzyme plasma (nonspecific) cholinesterase, usually after 3–5 min. A few people have abnormal plasma cholinesterase, and the action of suxamethonium may then last for hours or even days, during which time IPPV must continue without a break to allow the patient to survive. If treated in this way, the patient should eventually make a full recovery. No specific agent is available for reversing the action of suxamethonium.

If given in repeated doses, suxamethonium may cause bradycardia, and atropine should be given to prevent this. In patients with extensive tissue damage, for example a crush injury or severe burn, suxamethonium may lead to a massive loss of potassium ions from cells into the circulation and it is therefore contraindicated in such cases.

The commonest formulation of the drug is as liquid suxamethonium chloride in ampoules, but these must be kept refrigerated during transportation and storage, or activity will be lost. Powdered, heat-stable formulations of suxamethonium salts are available from a number of manufacturers. The bromide is slightly more potent than the chloride.

Non-depolarizing relaxants

These drugs block the acetylcholine receptors on the muscle but do not depolarize the muscle membrane. Their duration of action is usually around 30 min, which is longer than that of suxamethonium, and the onset is rather slower — up to 3 min for a full effect. An initial loading dose is normally followed by smaller increments, which maintain relaxation during surgery.

Neostigmine is used to antagonize the residual effect of non-depolarizing relaxants at the end of surgery. It is an acetylcholinesterase inhibitor and therefore causes an increase in the concentration of acetylcholine at the nerve endings. This acetylcholine antagonizes the muscle relaxant effects by competing with the relaxant drug for access to the receptors. If used alone, neostigmine would cause severe bradycardia (even cardiac arrest) and the production of copious secretions as a result of cholinergic stimulation of vagus nerve endings. It must therefore be given only with or immediately after atropine injected intravenously. Normal doses are atropine 0.02 mg/kg of body weight and neostigmine 0.04 mg/kg. The actions of non-depolarizing relaxants can be successfully reversed only after the effects have begun to wear off — at least 15 min after the last increment is given.

Many different non-depolarizing relaxants are available, but their actions are all basically similar. The two most commonly available are gallamine and alcuronium.

Gallamine is probably the most widely used in its class, and tends to produce a tachycardia by a vagolytic effect. Its excretion is entirely by the kidney, so it must not be given to patients with renal failure. The usual dose is 1–1.5 mg/kg of body weight, with increments of 0.5 mg/kg.

Alcuronium has little effect on the cardiovascular system and its actions can usually be reversed without difficulty. The usual dose is 0.2 mg/kg of body weight, with increments of 0.07 mg/kg.

Other non-depolarizing relaxants may be used if available. Curare, usually used in the form of tubocurarine, is fairly expensive, but is the established favourite of many; it causes marked histamine release and tends to reduce blood pressure. Pancuronium is a potent synthetic agent that has little effect on blood pressure, but it requires refrigerated storage. Atracurium and vecuronium are recent introductions claimed to have a short and predictable action that is rapidly reversible. Vecuronium has the advantage of being presented as a heat-stable powder with a shelf life of 3 years.

Guidelines and warnings for the use of relaxants

1. Never give a relaxant to a patient whose airway may be difficult to manage.

2. Always allow the effects of suxamethonium to wear off before giving a dose of another relaxant.

3. Never attempt to reverse the effects of a non-depolarizing relaxant before evidence of a return of muscle tone or breathing in the patient.

4. Always give reversal agents if non-depolarizing relaxants have been used, even if their effects seem to have worn off.

5. Always remember that a relaxant is not an anaesthetic; check that you are keeping the patient properly asleep, or he or she may be merely paralysed, awake, and terrified.

6. Before extubation your patient must:

   - be capable of sustained muscular contraction, for example of raising the head or limbs against the force of gravity;

   - be turned into the lateral position (unless there is a specific reason for not doing so).

10
Conduction anaesthesia

General anaesthesia relies on the action of drugs within the central nervous system to produce unconsciousness and depress responses to painful stimulation. Techniques of conduction (regional) anaesthesia use locally acting drugs to block nerve impulses before they reach the central nervous system.

Local anaesthetic drugs depress the electrical excitability of tissues (hence also their use to treat cardiac dysrhythmias). When injected close to nerve axons to give a high local concentration, such drugs block the passage of the depolarization wave necessary for the transmission of nerve impulses. The slenderest fibres (which carry the sensations of pain and temperature, and also efferent sympathetic impulses) are blocked first, those carrying touch and proprioception impulses next, and motor fibres (which control muscle tone as well as voluntary movement) last of all. A high concentration of drug will block all sensation and movement, while a low concentration will block only pain sensation, producing a "differential block". Differential block can almost always be observed during the onset and recovery periods of a successful block — the sensations of pinprick and temperature disappear first and are regained last. The onset of a successful block is often shown by the vasodilatation resulting from sympathetic blockade.

Toxicity and safety of local anaesthetic drugs

All local anaesthetic drugs are potentially toxic. The absorption of a large dose produces depression of the central nervous system with drowsiness, which may progress to unconsciousness with twitching and possibly convulsions. There may be hypotension related either to extensive sympathetic blockade, for example after "high" spinal anaesthesia, or to direct myocardial depression from high blood levels of the drug. These reactions are most likely to occur if the drug is accidentally injected into a vein or if an overdose is given by using either too high a concentration or too large a volume of drug. Toxic effects — usually cardiac dysrhythmias — may also occur after intravascular injection or rapid absorption of a vasoconstrictor drug such as epinephrine, which is frequently mixed with local anaesthetic to prolong the latter's action. Occasionally, patients have a true allergic reaction to the local anaesthetic drug, but this is unusual.

If a severe toxic reaction occurs, prompt resuscitation is needed; give oxygen and IPPV if there is severe respiratory depression. Convulsions, when associated with hypoxia, are best treated initially by giving a dose of suxamethonium and ventilating the lungs. If the convulsions persist, you may need to give anticonvulsant drugs such as diazepam or thiopental intravenously, but they should not be given as first-line treatment to a patient who may be hypotensive. It follows from the above that *full facilities for resuscitation should be available whenever you use conduction anaesthesia,* just as they should when you use general anaesthesia.

Safe and toxic doses

As with all drugs, the maximum safe dose is related to the size and condition of the patient. Blood levels (which reflect systemic absorption) tend to be higher when more concentrated solutions are used; for example, 5 ml of a 2% lidocaine solution (20 mg/ml) will produce higher blood levels than 10 ml of a 1% solution. Avoid toxicity by using the most dilute solution that will do the job, for example 1% lidocaine or 0.25% bupivacaine for most nerve blocks and 0.5% lidocaine for simple infiltration. The rate of absorption of the drug can also be reduced by injecting it together with a vasoconstrictor drug such as epinephrine, which is most often used in a dilution of 5 μg/ml (1:200 000); for infiltration, 2.5 μg/ml (1:400 000) is enough. Pre-mixed ampoules of local anaesthetic and epinephrine are often available, but if not, you can easily make a 5 μg/ml dilution by adding 0.1 ml of a 0.1% epinephrine solution to 20 ml of local anaesthetic solution. The addition of epinephrine has two useful effects: it reduces the rate at which local anaesthetic is absorbed from the injection site (by causing vasoconstriction) and therefore allows a larger dose of local anaesthetic to be used without toxic effects; at the same time, since local anaesthetic is removed from the injection site more slowly, the duration of anaesthesia increases by up to 50%. Epinephrine and other vasoconstrictor drugs must never be used for parts of the body that do not have a collateral circulation (ears, fingers, toes, and penis) as they could produce ischaemic damage, nor of course should they be used for intravenous regional anaesthesia.

Table 2. Maximum safe doses of local anaesthetic drugs

Drug	Maximum dose (mg/kg of body weight)	Maximum dose for 60-kg adult (ml)
Lidocaine 1%	4	24
Prilocaine 1%	6	36
Lidocaine 1% + epinephrine 5 μg/ml (1:200 000)	7	42
Bupivacaine 0.25%	1.5	36
Bupivacaine 0.25% + epinephrine 5 μg/ml (1:200 000)	2	48

The maximum safe doses of various local anaesthetic drugs are shown in Table 2. Note that for a 3-kg infant the toxic dose of 1% lidocaine is only 1.2 ml.

Contraindications to conduction anaesthesia

It is a common misconception that general anaesthesia is more dangerous than conduction anaesthesia. In fact, for major surgery, there is no evidence of any difference in morbidity and mortality between patients undergoing well-conducted general anaesthesia and those undergoing conduction anaesthesia. Certain specific contraindications to conduction anaesthesia exist, including the following:

- true allergy to local anaesthetic drugs
- sepsis at the intended site of injection
- inability to guarantee sterile equipment for injection
- systemic treatment of the patient with anticoagulant drugs (though local infiltration of a local anaesthetic drug on a small scale is permissible).

Other, but not absolute, contraindications include reluctance of the patient to undergo conduction anaesthesia, "difficult" sites of operation, and prolonged surgical procedures. In many cases, these last difficulties can be overcome by combining conduction anaesthesia with intravenous sedation or with light general anaesthesia.

General precautions and basic equipment

Before beginning any form of conduction anaesthesia, you should:

- ensure that the patient has been properly prepared and fasted as for general anaesthesia, which may become necessary if the conduction anaesthesia is unsuccessful;
- ensure that apparatus for resuscitation is at hand in case there is an adverse reaction;
- insert an indwelling needle or cannula and, for major operations, set up an intravenous infusion of an appropriate fluid.

Specimen techniques

Practical conduction anaesthesia cannot be learned from a book, but only by working with an experienced practitioner. There are many hundreds of individual conduction anaesthetic techniques and few anaesthetists would claim to be expert in all of them. The specimen techniques described here are intended as a reminder of the important aspects of a few useful techniques that should have already been demonstrated for you. Epidural anaesthetic techniques have been deliberately omitted since they generally require more skill and experience, are more difficult, take longer to perform, and are less predictable in their effects than the alternative, which is usually a (subarachnoid) spinal anaesthetic technique.

In the description of each technique it is assumed that the site of injection has been thoroughly cleaned and then prepared with a bactericidal antiseptic.

Topical anaesthesia of mucous membranes

This can be performed very simply by applying 4% lidocaine (or 5% cocaine if available) to the mucous membrane. It is suitable for instrumentation and minor operations on the nose, and superficial surgical procedures on the eye. Topical anaesthesia of the mouth, pharynx, and larynx is also possible and is one of the methods recommended for use in a patient whose airway is or may be difficult to manage, but do not anaesthetize the larynx if the stomach is full, as this will remove the patient's protective reflexes and make regurgitation likely. The simplest way to anaesthetize the larynx is to insert a 21-gauge needle through the cricothyroid membrane into the lumen of the trachea, where you should be able to aspirate air freely (Fig. 10.1), then rapidly inject 3 ml of 4% lidocaine, and remove the needle instantly (the patient will cough). Spray the throat with another 2 ml of 4% lidocaine, and after a few minutes laryngoscopy and intubation will be possible. Extreme gentleness and a gradual approach are necessary.

Simple infiltration

For infiltration you will need a sterile syringe with a fine needle and lidocaine 0.5% with epinephrine 5 μg/ml (1:200 000) or, if a large volume is needed, lidocaine 0.375% with epinephrine 3.3 μg/ml (1:300 000). If necessary, you can use up to 120 ml of the weaker concentration in a normal 65-kg adult.

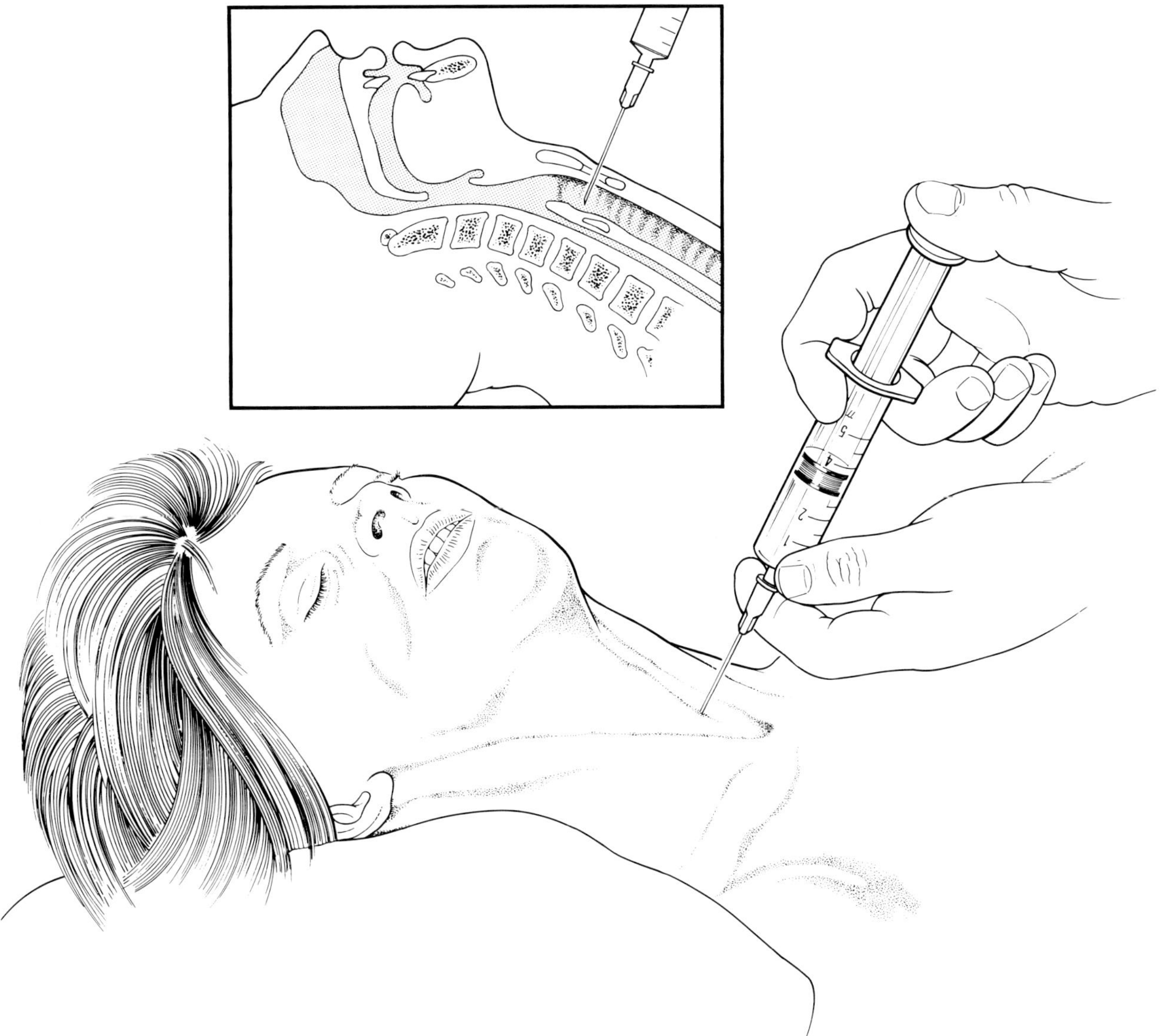

Fig. 10.1. Local anaesthesia of the larynx by cricothyroid injection.

For suturing a wound, after skin preparation with antiseptic, inject the local anaesthetic solution superficially (where most of the nerve endings are) about 5 mm from the margins of the wound, and allow about 5 min for the block to take effect.

Field blocks

The principle of a field block is to lay down a "barrage" of local anaesthetic to block all the sensory nerves that supply the operation site. It is particularly useful for areas where the nerve supply is both complex and variable, the groin for example, and can also be used for caesarean section if other methods of anaesthesia are not possible.

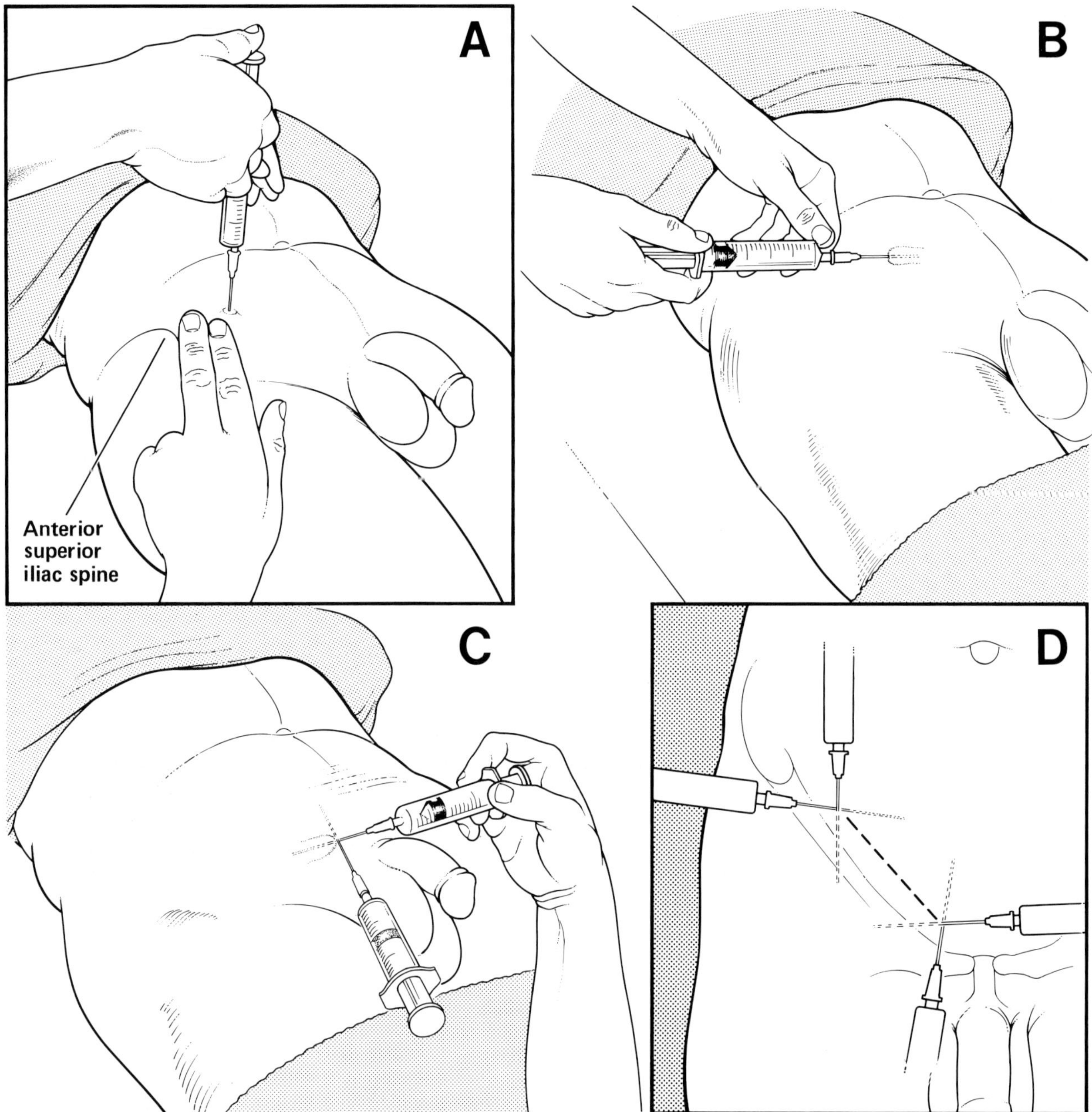

Fig. 10.2. Stages in performing an inguinal field block.

For repair of an inguinal hernia

Lidocaine 1.0% with epinephrine is used for this block. From a point two fingers' breadth from the anterior superior iliac spine, infiltrate the muscles in front of the pelvis with 5 ml of solution (Fig 10.2A). Use a long, fine needle to avoid multiple punctures, and keep the point of the needle moving during injection to avoid accidentally injecting a significant amount into any vessel. From the same point, inject 5 ml medially under the external oblique aponeurosis, directing the point of the needle towards the midline (Fig. 10.2B). From a second injection point above the pubic tubercle, infiltrate 5 ml under the external oblique aponeurosis with the needle directed towards the umbilicus and another 5 ml in the same plane in a lateral direction (Fig. 10.2C). Finally, inject about 5 ml "fan-wise" in the subcutaneous plane from each end of the planned line of the incision (Fig. 10.2D). If the hernia is reducible, inject 5 ml more into the superficial inguinal ring at the midpoint of the inguinal ligament. If necessary, further injection can be made by the surgeon into the deeper tissues during the operation. Field block does not of course anaesthetize any bowel or intraperitoneal tissue, which the surgeon should therefore handle gently.

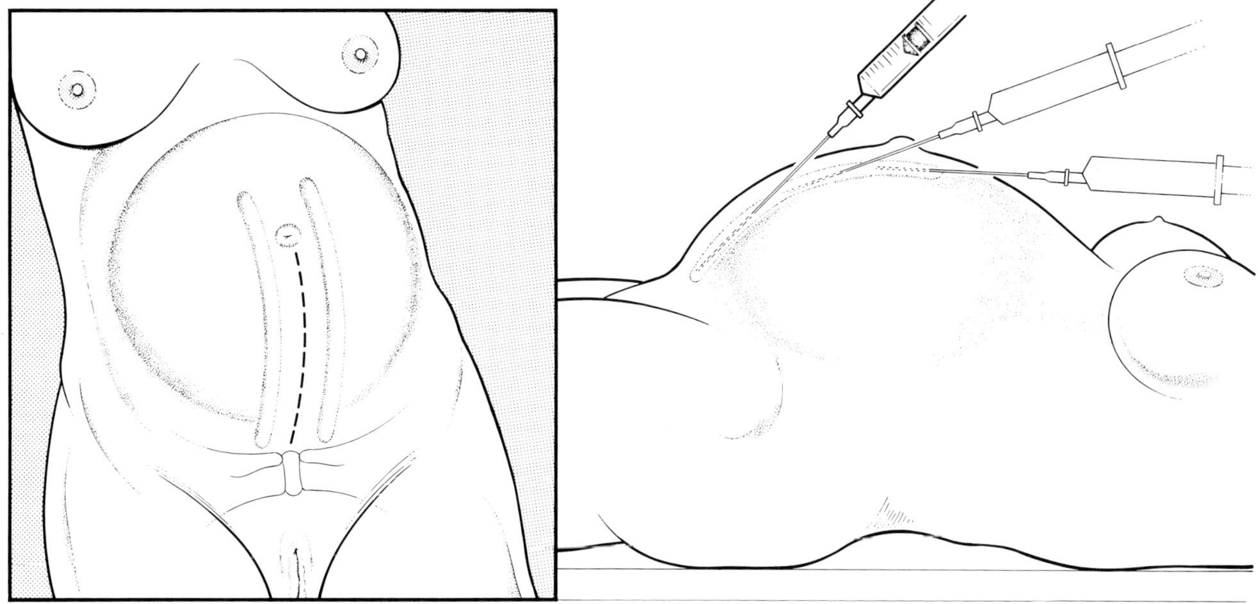

Fig. 10.3. Field block for caesarean section.

For caesarean section

A long wheal of local anaesthetic solution is raised 3–4 cm either side of the midline from the symphysis pubis to a point 5 cm above the umbilicus (Fig. 10.3). Infiltrate the solution down through the layers of the abdominal wall using a long needle, which should remain almost parallel to the skin. Be careful not to pierce the peritoneum and insert the needle into the uterus, as the abdominal wall is very thin at term. Up to 100 ml of 0.5% lidocaine with epinephrine may be used. The procedure may be uncomfortable for the mother, but analgesics and sedatives must not be given intravenously or the baby's physiological functions will be depressed. However, the inhalation of trichloroethylene 0.3–0.5% or nitrous oxide 50% in oxygen is safe (oxygen should, in any case, be given if available). Once the baby is delivered, you can of course give opiates intravenously to the mother to make her more comfortable.

For circumcision

Inject a ring of local anaesthetic (without epinephrine) subcutaneously and intradermally around the base of the penis; block each dorsal nerve by an injection of 5 ml into the dorsum of the penis, with the needle resting against the corpus cavernosum (Fig. 10.4A). Block the para-urethral branches by injecting ventrally, with the penis pulled up, into the grooves between the corpora cavernosum and spongiosum (Fig. 10.4B,C,D).

Nerve block techniques

The aim here is to deposit local anaesthetic next to a specified nerve to block sensation from the area that it innervates. The concentration of anaesthetic used (1% lidocaine or occasionally 1.5–2%) is slightly higher than for field block, which largely affects the nerve endings, as the drug may have to diffuse through a fibrous nerve sheath.

Digital nerve block (ring block)

Each digit is supplied by two dorsal and two palmar/plantar branches of the digital nerve, which can be simply blocked by a ring of local anaesthetic injected at the base of the digit (Fig. 10.5). A tourniquet is applied to localize the anaesthetic and to minimize bleeding. Do not use more than 4 ml of solution (1% lidocaine) per digit, or the tissues may be damaged by the high pressure developed. *Epinephrine must never be used in ring blocks.*

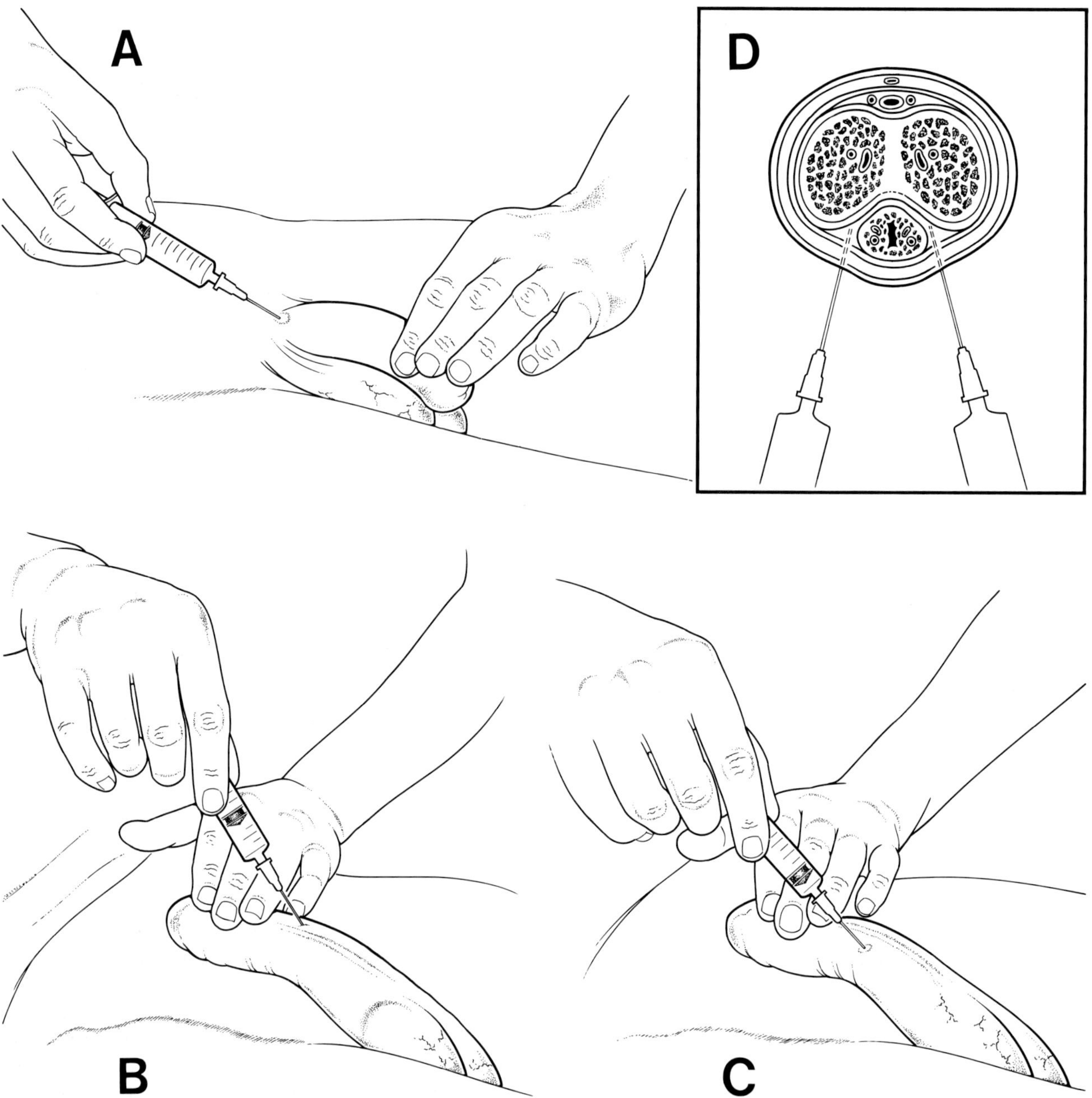

Fig. 10.4. Field block for circumcision. (A) Injection to block the dorsal nerves; (B,C,D) injection to block the para-urethral branches.

Nerve block at the ankle

Three separate injections are needed for this useful block, so it is kind to give the patient some basal sedation or analgesia or both. The anterior tibial nerve is first anaesthetized with 2–3 ml of 1% lidocaine injected on the anterior surface of the tibia at a point midway between the malleoli (Fig. 10.6A). The posterior tibial nerve is then blocked by an injection midway between the medial malleolus and the Achilles tendon: advance the needle perpendicular to the skin until bone is contacted; then withdraw slightly and inject 2 ml of 1% lidocaine (Fig. 10.6B). Thirdly, block the terminal branches of the saphenous and sural nerves by subcutaneous infiltration of up to 10 ml of solution along a line joining the malleoli around the front of the ankle (Fig. 10.6C,D).

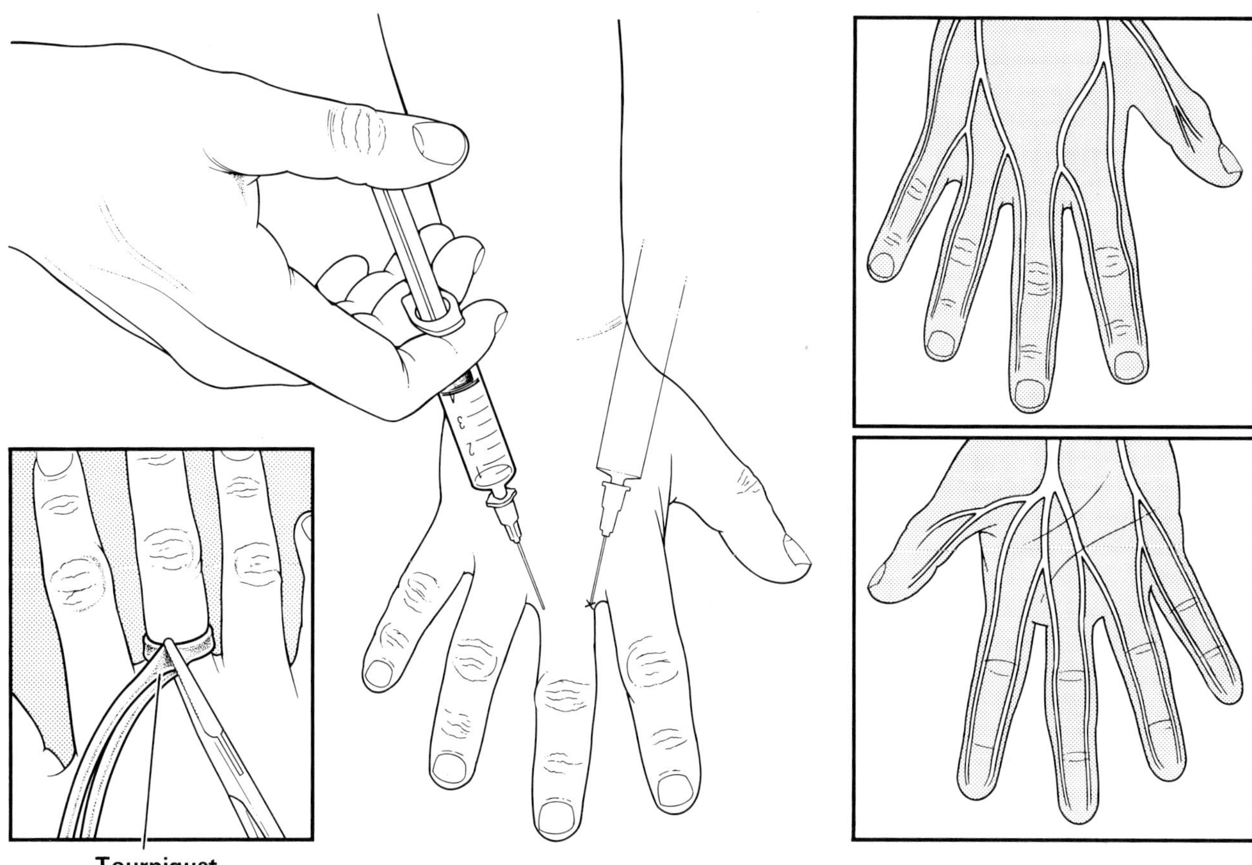

Fig. 10.5. Digital nerve block: injection at the base of the digit to block the dorsal and palmar branches of the nerve. (This block can also be used for the toes.)

Axillary block of the brachial plexus

The lower part of the brachial plexus is contained within a fibrous sheath, which also carries the axillary artery and vein. The nerve tissue is in three bundles, or cords, described as medial, posterior, and lateral in relation to the artery. Injection of local anaesthetic into this sheath is capable of producing conduction anaesthesia of the upper limb (except for the area innervated by the musculocutaneous nerve, which leaves the main nerve bundle rather high in the axilla). When performed successfully, this block allows surgery on most of the upper limb, and the use of a tourniquet when required.

Ask the patient to lie supine with the arm to be anaesthetized positioned to produce 90 degrees of abduction and external rotation (a suitable position is with the patient's hand under his or her head). Palpate the axillary artery and, after skin preparation, insert a short needle just above or below the artery (Fig. 10.7). You may feel the needle enter the sheath, and the patient may report tingling in the arm. When the needle is correctly placed (do not attach the syringe yet), you will see it move with every pulsation of the artery. If you insert the needle into the artery or vein by accident, remove it and apply firm pressure for 3 min; provided that a haematoma does not occur, you can then make another attempt. Once the needle is correctly placed, connect the syringe and inject 30 ml of 1% lidocaine with epinephrine. You must be absolutely certain before you do this that the needle is not in a vessel. If your needle is correctly placed, the patient may again report tingling. A correctly placed injection does not cause a large swelling, as the local anaesthetic solution is carried upwards in the sheath towards the neck. During injection, your assistant should press firmly on the artery about 3 cm below the point of injection to compress the sheath and prevent local anaesthetic from passing down the arm, where it would be wasted.

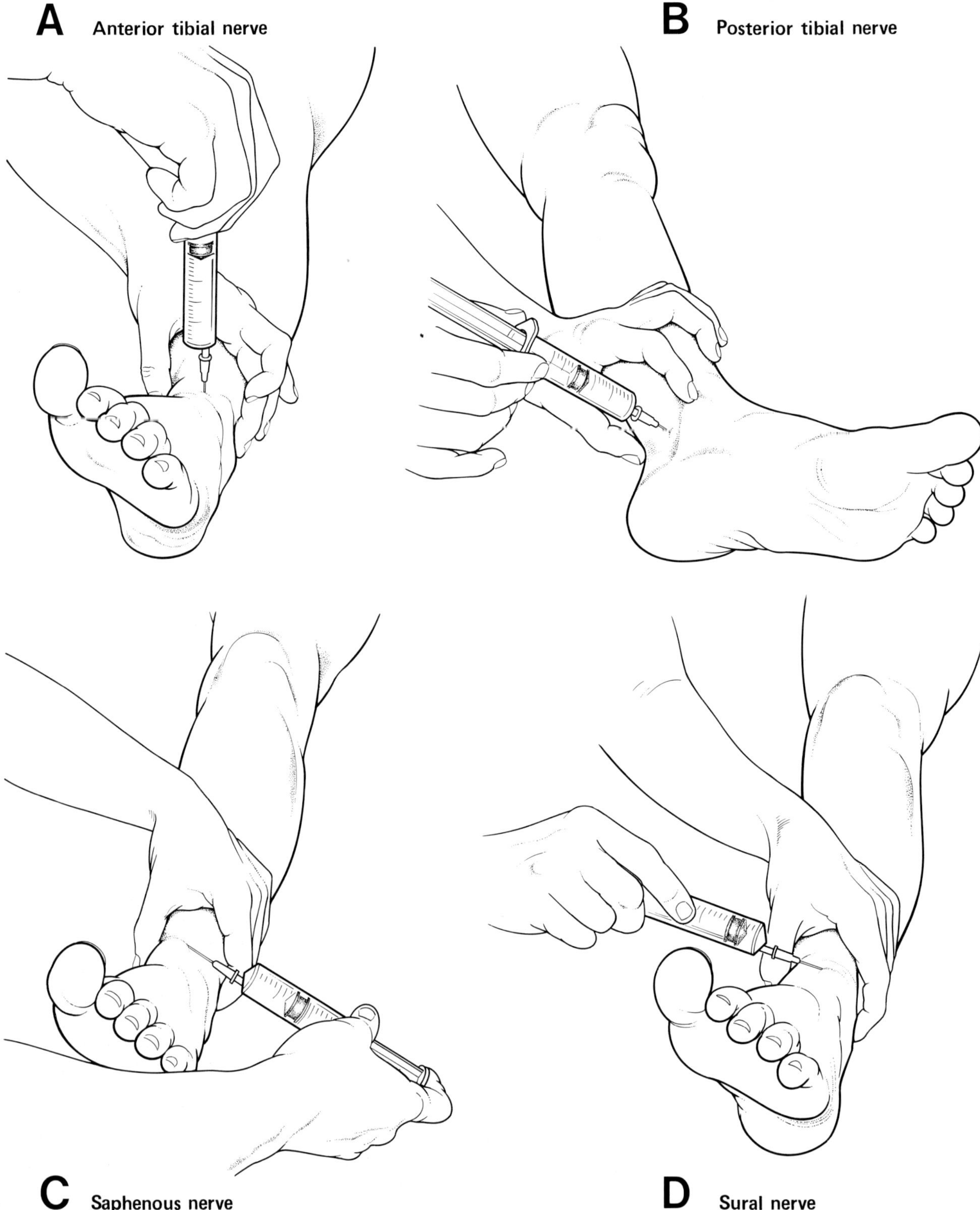

Fig. 10.6. Nerve block at the ankle.

As an alternative to digital pressure, some anaesthetists prefer to apply a light tourniquet below the injection site. The commonest mistake with this block is to inject too deeply; the sheath is superficial in position, often only 2–3 mm from the skin. After injection, the block develops slowly and may take up to 30 min to become effective. If bupivacaine has been used, the block can last for up to 12 hours, providing good postoperative pain relief. Bupivacaine is not, however, suitable for outpatient treatment, since a patient should not be sent home with a numb, paralysed arm.

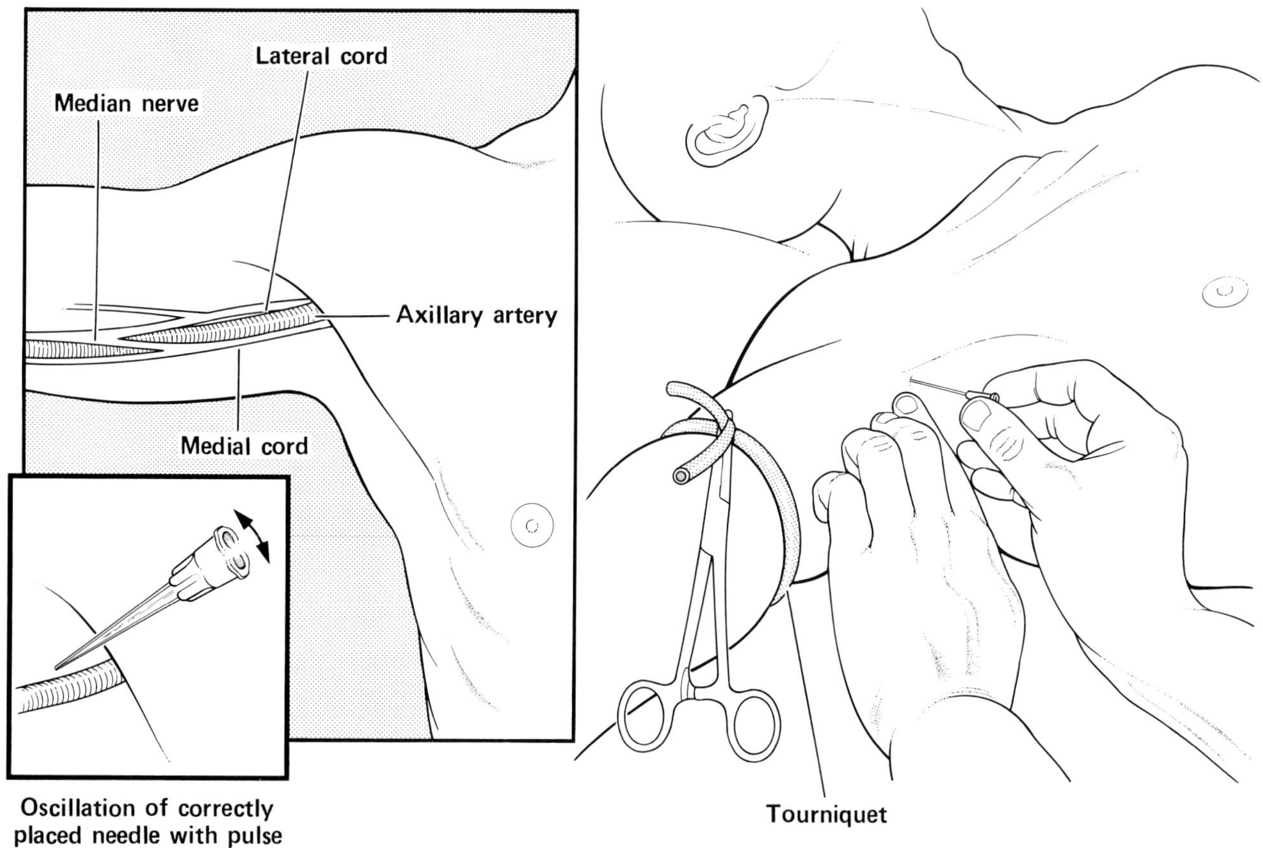

Fig. 10.7. Axillary block of the brachial plexus.

Block of the inferior alveolar nerve (dental block)

This block is suitable for certain dental procedures on the lower jaw. The inferior alveolar nerve runs inferiorly along the medial surface of the mandibular ramus and is blocked at a point just before it enters the mandibular foramen at the lingula. With the patient's mouth wide open, insert a needle just medial to the anterior border of the mandible, inside the mouth, at a point 1 cm above the occlusal (biting) surface of the lower third molar (Fig. 10.8). With the barrel of the syringe lying over the lower premolar teeth on the opposite side, slowly advance the needle, injecting a little local anaesthetic solution as you do so, keeping the syringe parallel to the floor of the mouth. After advancing approximately 2 cm, the needle will come into contact with bone. Withdraw it a fraction to prevent discomfort to the patient and slowly inject 2 ml of 2% lidocaine with epinephrine. Most oral surgeons prefer to use 12.5 μg/ml epinephrine solutions (1:80 000) if available, as 5 μg/ml solutions (1: 200 000) are rather short-acting. If required, block of the lingual nerve may be achieved by withdrawing the needle approximately 1 cm and slowly injecting a further 1 ml of local anaesthetic solution.

Intercostal nerve block

This block can be used to provide excellent pain relief for patients with fractured ribs; it can also provide worthwhile relaxation of the anterior abdominal wall during abdominal surgery. For alleviating the pain of a fractured rib, it is obviously necessary to block the nerve of the rib concerned. For analgesia or relaxation of the abdominal wall, the intercostal nerves of the dermatomes in the region of the proposed operation need to be blocked. (The dermatome supplied by the sixth intercostal nerve is at the level of the xiphisternum, that supplied by the tenth at about the level of the umbilicus, and that supplied by the twelfth in the suprapubic region.)

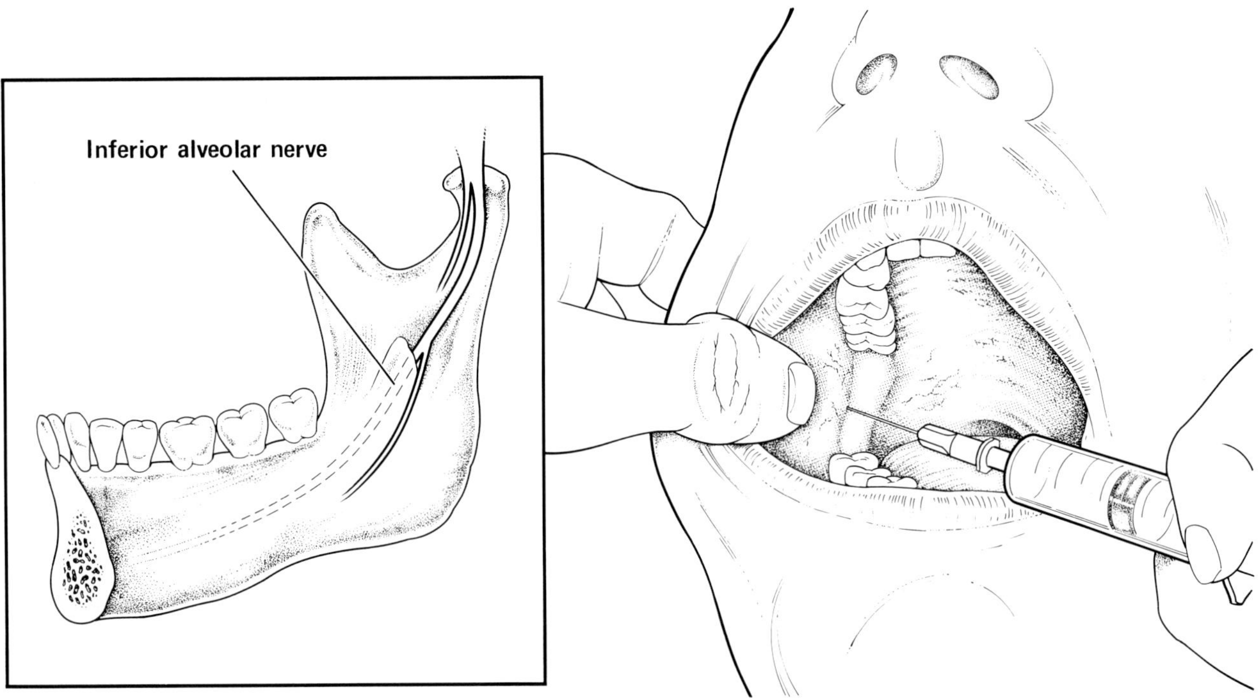

Fig. 10.8. Block of the inferior aveolar nerve.

For abdominal relaxation and analgesia, the nerves can conveniently be blocked in the mid-axillary line, but for fractures the block should be more posterior, preferably close to the angle of the rib (Fig. 10.9).

Each intercostal nerve runs parallel to the lower border of its rib in the intercostal groove, just below the intercostal artery and vein. To allow you to reach the posterior part of the rib, the patient should sit up with both arms folded over a pillow in order to move the scapula laterally and give access to the upper ribs. For the approach in the mid-axillary line, the patient can lie supine with the arm abducted. In either case, palpate the rib, and after making a small skin wheal level with the lower border of the rib, advance the needle slowly until it makes contact with bone. Inject a small amount of local anaesthetic (the periosteum is sensitive), and then "walk" the needle slowly down the rib in a caudal direction until it slips off the lower edge (Fig. 10.9). Advance the needle another 2–3 mm (but no more, as the pleura is close) and inject 2.5 ml of local anaesthetic — lidocaine 1% with epinephrine or bupivacaine 0.25% with or without epinephrine. Repeat the procedure on as many ribs as necessary, but be careful not to exceed the maximum dose of anaesthetic. Pneumothorax is a potential but rare complication of this block, so watch the patient carefully afterwards.

Femoral nerve block

This block can be used for surgery on the front of the thigh, but its main use is to provide excellent analgesia for the patient with a fractured femoral shaft. It is extremely useful when such a patient must be transported.

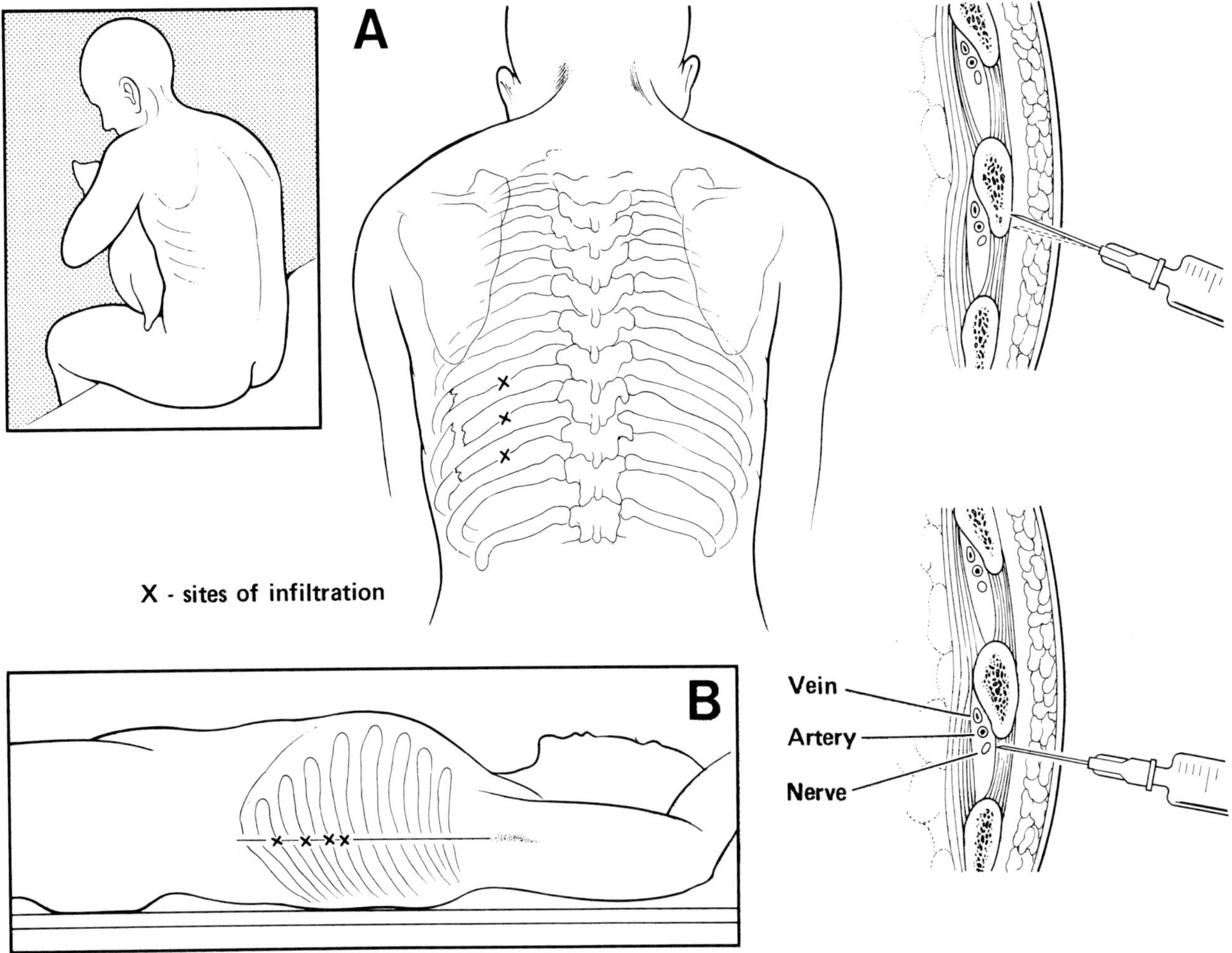

Fig. 10.9. Intercostal nerve block. (A) Suggested approach for rib fractures; (B) suggested approach for abdominal relaxation.

The femoral nerve passes under the inguinal ligament and lies lateral to the femoral artery. Block it by injecting 15 ml of 1% lidocaine into the arterial sheath (as in an axillary block) just below the inguinal ligament and lateral to the artery. Having done this, inject a further 5 ml subcutaneously, moving laterally, to block any high branches of the nerve (Fig. 10.10).

Intravenous regional anaesthesia

This technique consists of the intravenous injection of local anaesthetic drug into an arm that is isolated from the circulation by an arterial tourniquet. The technique provides good analgesia, but, because of the progressive discomfort caused by the tourniquet, its use should be limited to procedures lasting less then one hour. Sudden collapse of the patient is always a possibility and may occur if local anaesthetic drug escapes beneath the tourniquet during injection or when the tourniquet is released at the end of surgery. Full resuscitation apparatus must therefore be available.

To ensure venous access at all times, insert a cannula or needle into a vein on the side of the patient opposite the side of the proposed operation. Next, cannulate a vein in the arm to be anaesthetized and exsanguinate the arm either with an Esmarch bandage or, in the case of a fracture, by simply elevating the arm for 3 min. Apply a proper arterial tourniquet (a blood pressure cuff will *not* do) and inflate it to 100 mmHg (13.3 kPa) above the patient's systolic blood pressure. Through the cannula in the isolated arm inject 20–40 ml of prilocaine 0.5% or lidocaine 0.5% (*without* epinephrine). Do *not* use higher concentrations or bupivacaine as these can be fatal if given intravenously. Analgesia begins in a few

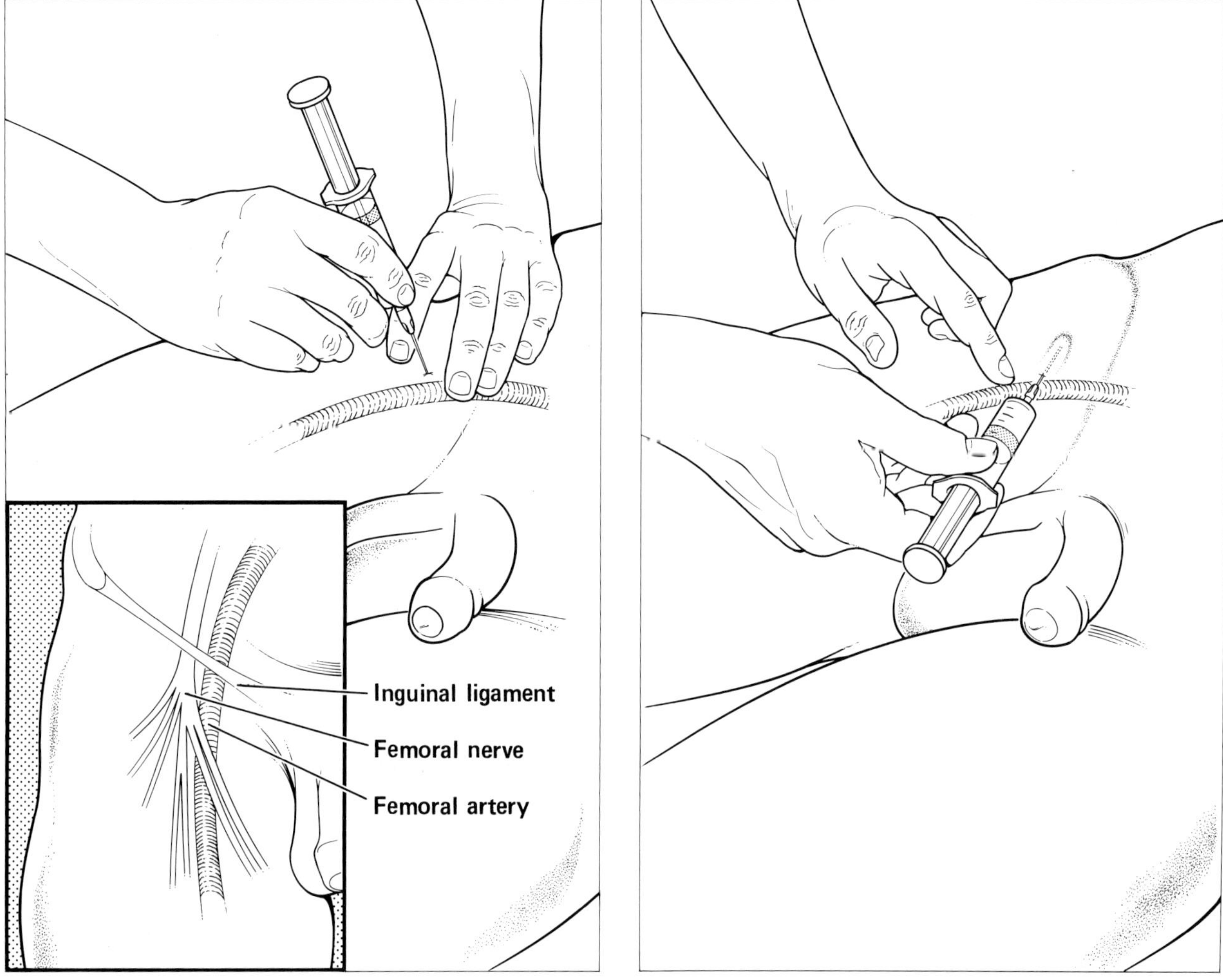

Fig. 10.10. Femoral nerve block.

minutes and will last as long as the tourniquet remains inflated. However short the procedure, always leave the tourniquet inflated *for at least 20 min* to allow some of the local anaesthetic to become fixed to the tissues and to prevent systemic blood levels of the drug becoming dangerously high after release of the tourniquet.

Spinal anaesthesia

In spinal anaesthesia, a conduction block of nerve roots is achieved by injecting a small volume of concentrated local anaesthetic solution into the subarachnoid space through a lumbar puncture. Injection is made at a level below that of the first lumbar vertebra (the level at which the spinal cord terminates), frequently at the interspace between the third and fourth lumbar vertebrae. A solution denser than cerebrospinal fluid is normally used, for example 5% lidocaine in 7.5% glucose ("heavy" lidocaine), which allows the nature of the block to be controlled by positioning the patient so that the drug flows "downhill" to the segments that need to be blocked. For example, injection with the patient in the sitting position will result in a block of the sacral nerve roots; injection with the patient in the lateral position, if the position is maintained, will produce unilateral anaesthesia on the lower side.

Successful spinal anaesthesia always produces a considerable block of the sympathetic nerves, resulting in widespread vasodilatation and a fall in blood pressure, which may be dangerous. The best way to prevent such a fall is to infuse intravenously 0.5–1 litre of saline or Hartmann's solution (for an adult) before the spinal injection. The management of the patient whose blood pressure has fallen unacceptably, in spite of these precautions, is detailed on page 100.

Indications for spinal anaesthesia

Spinal anaesthesia can be used for almost any operation in the lower abdomen (including caesarean section), perineum, or leg. It gives very good relaxation, but the duration of anaesthesia with lidocaine is limited to about 90 min. If other drugs such as bupivacaine, cinchocaine, or tetracaine are available, the duration of anaesthesia can be extended to 2–3 hours.

Contraindications for spinal anaesthesia

1. Spinal anaesthesia is contraindicated in a patient with uncorrected or undercorrected hypovolaemia. When not anaesthetized, the hypovolaemic patient may be able to sustain a relatively normal blood pressure by extensive vasoconstriction, but the sympathetic blockade that accompanies spinal anaesthesia and overrides this reflex will produce severe cardiovascular collapse. In an emergency, general anaesthesia is usually safer.

2. A patient with severe uncorrected anaemia or heart disease should also not be given spinal anaesthesia, since if hypotension occurs the patient's condition could be worsened.

3. As for other local anaesthetic techniques, local sepsis and anticoagulant therapy are contraindications.

Specimen technique

As with all other conduction blocks, full resuscitation equipment and the necessary drugs must be available and checked before starting. Set up an intravenous infusion and "pre-load" the patient with 500 ml of physiological saline. (The blood pressure falls fairly rapidly after spinal anaesthesia at all but the lowest levels of the spine, so it is better to be slightly ahead with fluid therapy.) Position the patient carefully in the sitting or lateral position, with the lumbar spine well flexed. It is easier to do this if you ask the patient to flex his or her head on to the chest in addition to flexing the spine and hips. Your assistant will need to support and hold the patient in position. With a marker or ball-point pen, draw the outlines of the lumbar spinous processes on the skin to help you to visualize the spinal anatomy. Mark your proposed site of injection and scrub your hands more thoroughly than the surgeon. (The surgeon has only to avoid a wound infection in the patient; you have to avoid meningitis!) Put on sterile gloves and thoroughly prepare the skin over a wide area of the back; place sterile towels around the proposed site of injection in such a way that they will not fall down and obscure your view. Choose a needle between 20- and 23-gauge with a stylet; fine needles produce a lower incidence of postspinal headache, but are more difficult to use. Do not touch the shaft of the spinal needle, which should either be a sterile disposable one or have been autoclaved — boiling is inadequate.

Choose whichever interspace below the second lumbar vertebra feels easiest to penetrate; a line joining the iliac crests usually passes through the level of the fourth lumbar vertebra or the interspace between the third and fourth lumbar vertebrae (Fig. 10.11). Raise a skin wheal with local anaesthetic over the chosen space in the midline and insert the spinal needle through the skin, supraspinous ligament, interspinous ligament, and ligamentum flavum. The needle should stay in the midline, but will need to be directed slightly towards the head to pass through the interspace. If you strike bone superficially, it is probably the spine of the vertebra above, so make a new start 1 cm further down. If you strike bone deep, it is the vertebra below, and you will need to angle the needle more towards the head. If the ligaments are calcified, move 1 cm laterally from the midline and try again, aiming for the midline as you advance the needle gradually. Once the needle has passed through the ligamentum flavum, remove the stylet and advance slowly. You may feel the needle enter the dura, and cerebrospinal fluid will start to flow out of the needle (Fig. 10.11). If it does not, try rotating the needle through 90 degrees, as a nerve root may be lying across the bevel. Once cerebrospinal fluid flows, connect the syringe and inject your drug, ensuring that the needle does not move. A small aspiration of 0.1 ml of liquid at the end of injection confirms that the needle has remained in the cerebrospinal fluid.

To block the sacral roots only, for example for surgery of the perineum, inject 1 ml of 5% heavy lidocaine with the patient in the sitting position; the patient should then remain sitting for 3 min.

For a higher block, for example for surgery of the legs and abdomen below the umbilicus, inject 1.5 ml with the patient in the lateral position and lie him or her supine with a 5-degree head-down tilt and one pillow under the head.

Complications of spinal anaesthesia

A fall in blood pressure is common after spinal anaesthesia. It usually occurs in the first 10 min after injection, so measure the blood pressure every 2 min during this period. If systolic blood pressure falls below 75 mmHg (10 kPa), or if the patient has symptoms from any fall in blood pressure, you must act quickly to avoid renal, cardiac, or cerebral damage. Give the patient oxygen and increase the drip rate; you may need to give a litre of fluid to restore the blood pressure. If the heart rate is below 65 beats per minute, give atropine 0.5 mg intravenously. Also consider the use of a vasopressor drug such as ephedrine, 15–25 mg given intravenously and 15–25 mg intramuscularly. Very rarely, a "total spinal" block develops, with anaesthesia and paralysis of the whole body, in which case, you will have to intubate the patient and ventilate the lungs, as well as treat the severe hypotension. With this management, the patient should come to no harm, and the total spinal block will wear off in a couple of hours.

Headache in the postoperative period is a recognized complication of spinal anaesthesia. Spinal headache is typically worse on sitting or standing and disappears on lying down. It is frontal or occipital and is not associated with neck rigidity. It is caused by loss of cerebrospinal fluid from the brain through the dural puncture — the larger the hole, the greater the chance of headache. It can be prevented by keeping the patient flat (allow one pillow) for 24 hours. If the headache still appears when the patient gets up, keep the patient flat and give plenty of fluids orally (or intravenously if necessary) and simple analgesics. Continue this treatment for 24 hours after the headache disappears, at which time the patient can be mobilized.

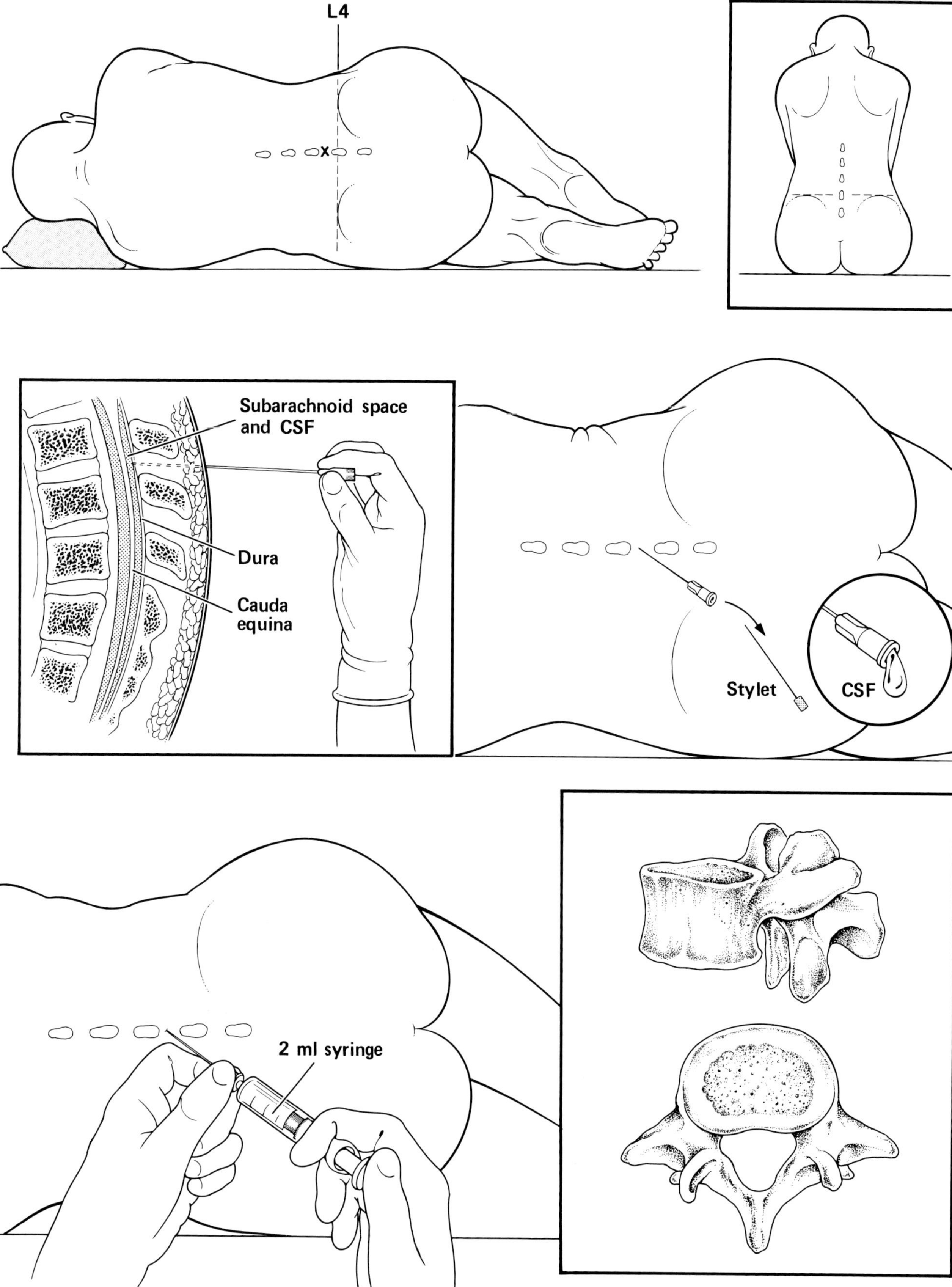

Fig. 10.11. Technique of spinal anaesthesia.

11
Choosing and planning your anaesthetic technique

In anaesthesia, as in most areas of medicine and surgery, you will need at least as much knowledge and skill to make the right choice of technique as you will to implement it. This book cannot tell you which anaesthetic to choose. The anaesthetic of choice in any given situation depends on your training and experience, the range of equipment and drugs available, and the clinical situation. One "golden rule" is worth remembering: *however strong the indications may seem for using a particular technique, especially in an emergency, the best anaesthetic technique will be one with which you are most experienced and confident.*

Some of the factors to bear in mind when choosing your anaesthetic technique are:

- training and experience of anaesthetist and surgeon
- availability of drugs and equipment
- medical condition of the patient
- time available
- emergency or elective procedure
- presence of a full stomach
- patient's preference.

Not all these factors are of equal importance, but all should be considered, especially when the choice of technique is not obvious.

Choice of anaesthetic technique for a particular operation

Table 3 is intended to help you decide what type of anaesthetic might be most suitable for a given surgical procedure. For minor emergency operations (for example the suture of a wound or manipulation of an arm fracture), when the patient probably has a full stomach, conduction (regional) anaesthesia is probably the wisest choice. For major emergency operations, there is often little difference in safety between conduction and general anaesthesia.

When you have come to a decision, discuss it with the surgeon and theatre team, who may give you further relevant information. For example, the proposed operation may need more time than can be provided by the technique you have suggested. Also check that you have all the drugs and equipment you may need.

Table 3. Suitable anaesthetic techniques for different types of surgery

Type of surgery	Suitable anaesthetic technique
Major head and neck surgery Upper abdominal Intrathoracic	General endotracheal
Lower abdominal Groin, perineum Lower limbs	General endotracheal *or* Spinal *or* Nerve or field block *or* Combined general and conduction
Upper limbs	General endotracheal *or* Nerve block *or* Intravenous regional

By now you will probably have decided, in principle, on one of the following techniques:

- general anaesthesia with drugs given intravenously or by inhalation
- spinal anaesthesia
- nerve block
- infiltration anaesthesia.

There can be advantages in combining light general anaesthesia with a conduction block because such a technique reduces the amount of general anaesthetic that the patient requires and allows a rapid recovery, with postoperative analgesia provided by the remaining conduction block.

Planning general anaesthesia

Fig. 11.1 shows the possibilities you should consider when planning general anaesthesia. The right-hand side of the diagram shows what is effectively a universal anaesthetic technique, which can be used for almost any operation and which you should master and practise regularly.

For general anaesthesia, endotracheal intubation should be routine, unless there is a specific reason to avoid it. Endotracheal intubation is the most basic of anaesthetic skills, and you should be able to do it confidently whenever necessary. In smaller hospitals, many of the operations are emergencies, and the lungs and lives of the patients are in danger if you do not protect them by this manoeuvre.

Remember that all relaxants are contraindicated prior to endotracheal intubation if the patient has an abnormality of the jaw or neck or if there is any other reason to think that laryngoscopy and intubation might be difficult.

If you find intubation unexpectedly difficult after giving the patient suxamethonium and you do not succeed in intubating within 30 s of starting laryngoscopy, you must restore oxygenation by ventilating the patient with a face mask for 10 good breaths. Make one more attempt, and if you are still unsuccessful after another 30 s, adopt the "Failed intubation drill" (see page 21).

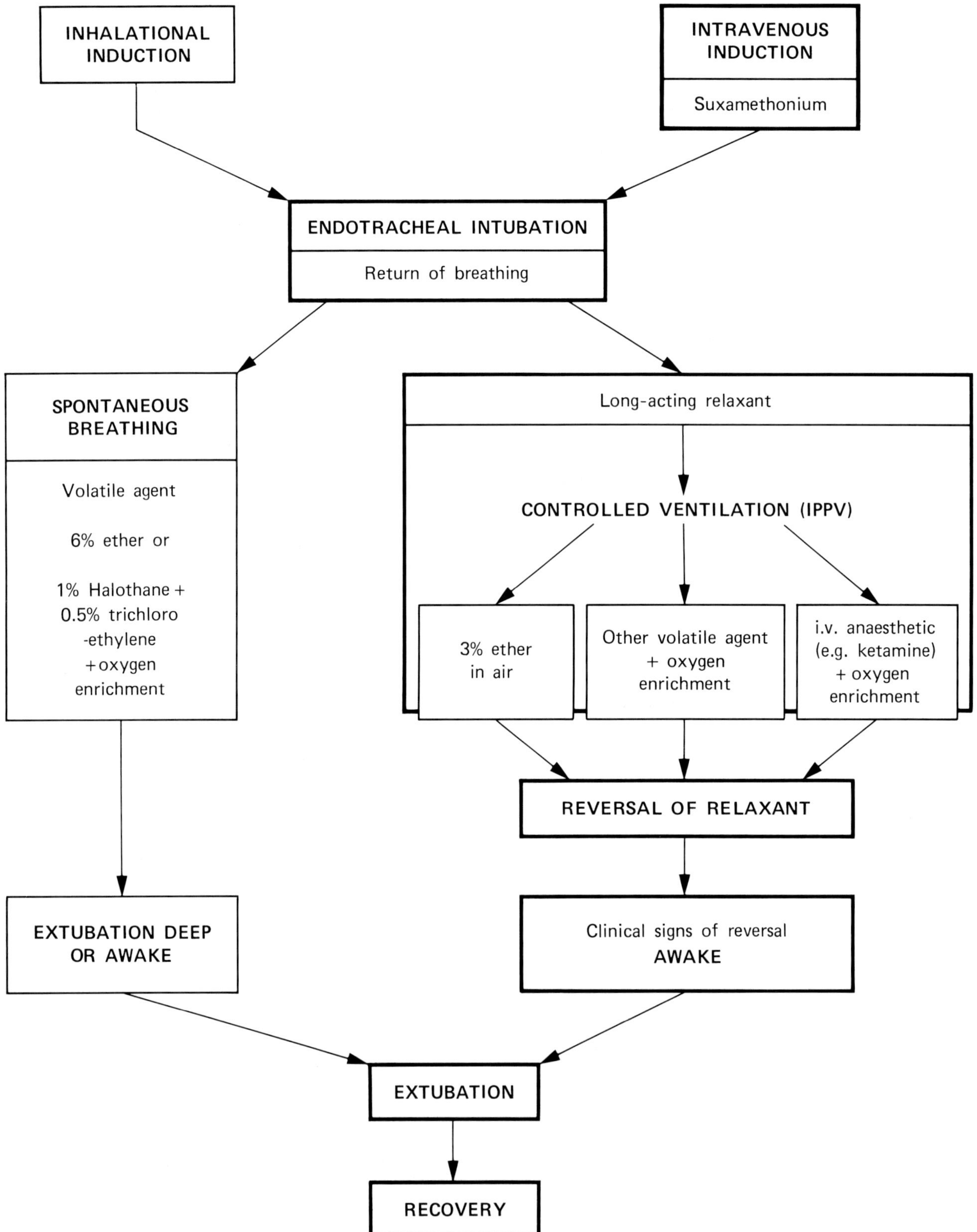

Fig. 11.1. Planning a general anaesthetic technique.

Safety of general and conduction techniques

In general, there are potential risks with all types of anaesthetic. These can be minimized, however, by careful assessment of the patient, thoughtful planning of the anaesthetic technique, and skilful performance by the anaesthetist. You should keep records of all the anaesthetics that you give (see Annex 3 for specimen chart) and regularly review complications and morbidity. Some of the possible complications to look for are listed in Table 4.

Table 4. Complications of general and conduction anaesthesia

General anaesthesia	Conduction anaesthesia
Airway obstruction	Toxicity of drug
Aspiration of gastric contents into the lungs	Accidental intravascular injection
Allergy or hypersensitivity	Allergic reactions
Hypotension (including supine hypotension in pregnancy)	Massive spread of spinal anaesthetic
Cardiac dysrhythmias	Cardiac depression by local anaesthetic drug
Trauma to mouth, pharynx, larynx, and teeth	Spread of sepsis
Respiratory depression	Depression of the central nervous system and convulsions
Increased intracranial pressure	
Postoperative hypoxia	
Toxic damage to liver or kidneys	

12
Postoperative care of the patient

As an anaesthetist, your responsibility includes the care of your patient while he or she is recovering from the effects of anaesthesia. Ensure that a trained nurse or assistant is available to observe the patient closely and make regular measurements of pulse rate, blood pressure, and respiratory rate, as well as to watch for and report any abnormal and continuing blood loss.

The first hour after anaesthesia is a potentially dangerous time for the patient. Protective airway reflexes are still depressed to some extent, even if the patient appears to be awake, and the residual effects of the drugs that you have given may lead to respiratory depression. Pain from the patient's wound, especially if it is in the upper abdomen or thorax, will prevent him or her from taking deep breaths or coughing effectively. This may lead to the development of a chest infection or collapse of the lung bases with further hypoxia. Patients who have not fully recovered consciousness should be nursed in the semiprone position, but patients with abdominal incisions, once fully awake, will usually find breathing easier in the reclining or sitting position. Oxygen may be given and should be routine for sick patients and for those who have had prolonged operations. The most economical way to give oxygen during recovery is with a soft nasopharyngeal catheter and a flow of 0.5–1.0 litres/min, which will usually produce a concentration of 30–40% oxygen in the inspired air. If the patient has pain, it should be controlled. If a strong, i.e., opiate, analgesic is needed, give the first dose intravenously, so that you can titrate the dose against the patient's pain and also observe any untoward respiratory depression. You can then prescribe the dose given intravenously for regular intramuscular use if required, with some confidence that analgesia will be adequate and the dosage safe.

Where should the patient recover?

Probably the safest place for the patient to recover is the operating theatre itself, since all necessary equipment and drugs are close by for access in the event of any mishap. It is often more convenient to move the patient out to a recovery area, so that the theatre can be cleaned and prepared for the next operation. Any recovery area must be clean, well lit, and near to the operating theatre so that you can visit the patient easily and quickly whenever needed. Effective suction apparatus should be available, as should an oxygen supply and resuscitation equipment. *Unconscious patients must never be sent back to the ward.*

You must see each patient before he or she leaves the recovery area and make a quick assessment by asking yourself the following questions:

- Does the patient have a good colour (mucous membranes, skin, etc.) when breathing air?
- Is the patient able to cough and maintain a clear airway?
- Is there any evidence of obstruction or laryngeal spasm?
- Can the patient lift his or her head from the bed for at least 3 s?

- Are the patient's pulse rate and blood pressure stable?
- Are the hands and feet warm and well perfused?
- Is there a good urinary output?
- Is the patient's pain controlled, and have necessary analgesics and fluids been prescribed?

Postoperative visiting and record-keeping

You should always visit your patient postoperatively on the ward to see whether any further treatment is necessary during recovery from the effects of anaesthesia. Keep a record (separate from the case notes) of the anaesthetic technique you used and of any complications. This will not only be of great interest to you in future, but will also help the next time you have a similar patient to anaesthetize. A good anaesthetist, however experienced, learns something from each case.

13
Paediatric and obstetric anaesthesia

Although the general principles of anaesthesia for adults outlined in this book are widely applicable, physiological differences in pregnant women and in children often make it necessary to use slightly different anaesthetic techniques for such patients and to take special care of them.

Anaesthesia for children

Most of the general principles of anaesthesia can be applied to children, but there are some significant anatomical and physiological differences between children and adults that can cause problems, especially in neonates and children weighing less than about 15 kg.

Anatomical differences and problems

The airway

A child has a large head in relation to body size and you must therefore position a child differently from an adult, sometimes with a pillow under the shoulders rather than the head, to clear the airway or to perform laryngoscopy (see Fig. 2.5, page 16). The larynx of a child also differs from that of an adult. In the adult the narrowest part of the air passage is at the level of the vocal cords; in the child the narrowest part is below this, at the level of the cricoid cartilage. The airway here is circular in cross-section, so a correct fit can usually be obtained with a plain (not cuffed) endotracheal tube. A small air leak should usually be present around the tube, but if a completely airtight fit is required, pack the pharynx with gauze moistened with water or saline; never use liquid paraffin (mineral oil), as this causes lung damage. Do not use a cuffed tube with an internal diameter less than 6.0 mm.

Because the airway of a child is narrow, a small amount of oedema can produce severe obstruction (Fig. 13.1). Oedema can easily be caused by forcing in an endotracheal tube that is too tight, so if you suspect that your tube is too large change it immediately. Damage is most likely from a tube that is both too large and left in the trachea too long. As a rough guide for normally nourished children more than about two years old, the internal diameter of the tube likely to be of the correct size can be calculated from the following formula, but you should always have one size larger and one smaller ready in case you need to change.

$$\text{Internal diameter (in mm)} = \frac{\text{Age (in years)}}{4} + 4.5$$

Another rough indicator of the correct size of tube is the diameter of the child's little finger. To estimate the length of tube needed, double the distance from the corner of the child's mouth to the ear canal; to check, look at the child's head from the side while holding the upper end of the tube level with the mouth to

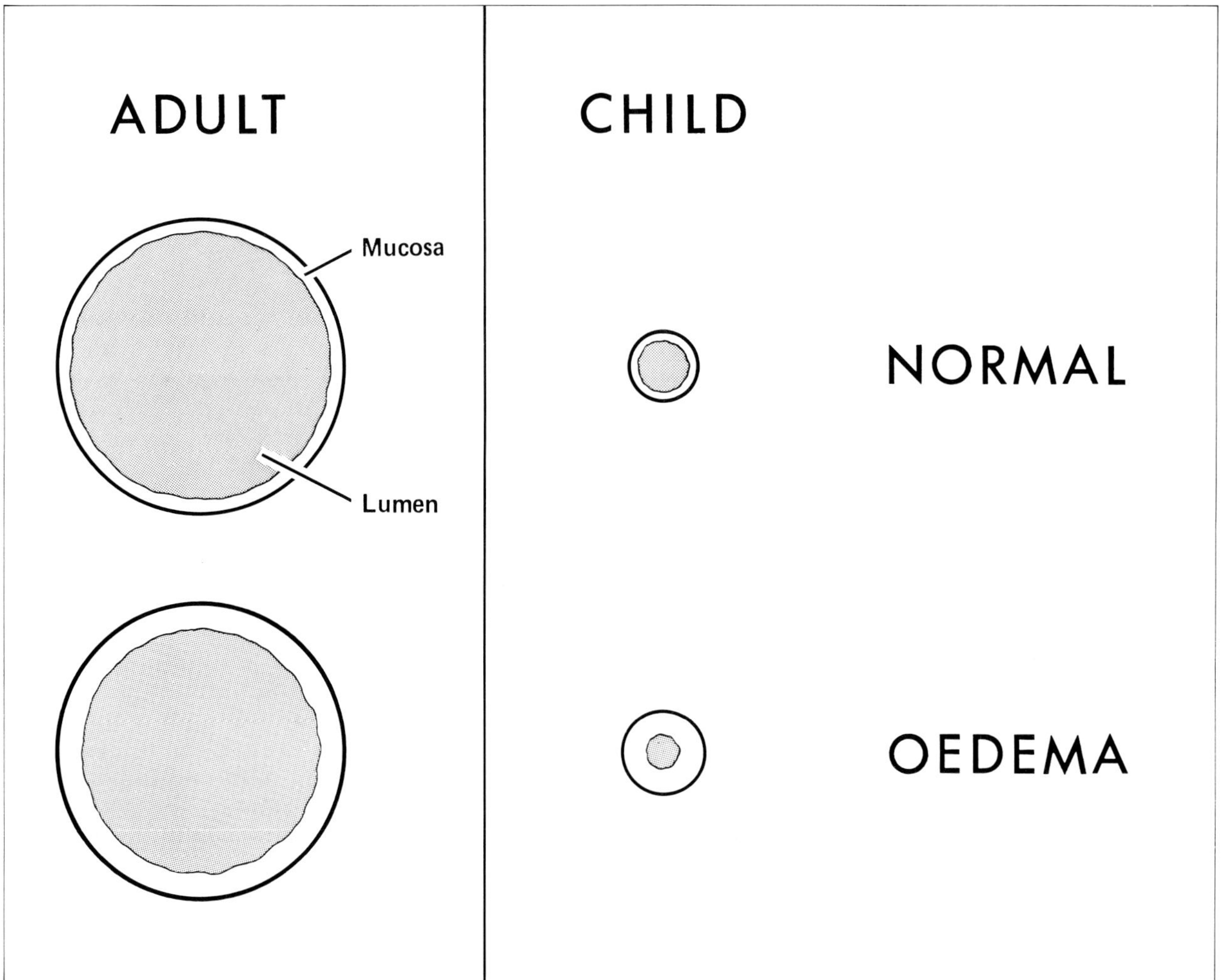

Fig. 13.1. The effects of mucosal oedema in the airway (shown in cross-section).

give you an idea of how far into the chest the tube will go. After intubation, always listen over both lungs to make sure that the tube has not entered a bronchus. Most neonates will need a tube of 3 mm internal diameter, though for premature infants a 2.5 mm tube may be necessary.

For intubating infants, many anaesthetists prefer to use a small straight laryngoscope blade (see Fig. 13.4, page 114). If one is not available, the tip of a Macintosh blade designed for adults can be used, as it is only slightly curved.

The abdomen

A child's abdomen is more protuberant than an adult's and contains the greater part of the viscera (many of the viscera of an adult are situated in the relatively larger pelvic cavity). The diaphragm is therefore less efficient in a child. The rib cage is also less rigid than an adult's. These factors mean that abdominal distension can very easily give rise to respiratory difficulty.

Physiological differences and problems

Metabolism and heart rate

The metabolic rate is higher in children than in adults, while the lungs are less efficient and smaller in relation to oxygen requirements. For this reason, children have higher respiratory rates than adults and their lungs must be ventilated more rapidly. Obstruction or apnoea leads to a very rapid onset of cyanosis. The heart rate is also higher than that of an adult, but the resting sympathetic tone is low, so reflex vagal stimulation can lead to severe bradycardia, for example during laryngoscopy or surgery. For this reason, atropine (0.015 mg/kg of body weight) is almost always included in premedication for infants.

Hypothermia

Hypothermia can occur very rapidly in an infant because of the high surface-to-volume ratio of the body; it may result in a severe metabolic disturbance. Take active steps to prevent hypothermia in any operating theatre with an ambient temperature below 26 °C. Carefully wrap the infant, including the head, which is a major source of heat loss; warm up antiseptic solutions before use on the skin; and protect the infant from draughts.

Hypoglycaemia

Hypoglycaemia may be a problem in babies. They do not need to be starved for more than 3 hours preoperatively and should be fed as soon as possible after the operation. Glucose infusions should be used during anaesthesia to help to maintain the blood sugar level. Infusing glucose instead of physiological saline also avoids a sodium load that the baby's kidneys are unable to excrete.

Circulation

The normal heart rate at birth is about 140 per minute, but it may swing widely in response to stress. The neonate has a proportionately higher blood volume (90 ml/kg of body weight) than the adult (70 ml/kg), but even so, what appears to be a small blood loss may have visible effects. Blood losses during the operation must be measured as accurately as possible. If suction apparatus is in use, a simple method is to use a measuring cylinder in the suction line rather than the usual large container. If blood loss amounts to more than 5% of blood volume, an intravenous infusion is necessary; if losses exceed 10% of blood volume, blood transfusion is indicated. For most paediatric operations, other than minor ones, it is routine to give glucose 5% (or glucose 4%, saline 0.18%) at a rate of 5 ml/kg of body weight per hour in addition to replacing the measured fluid losses.

Technical problems

Most children weighing more than 15 kg can be anaesthetized by using the techniques described in this book for adult patients, but with the dosage reduced in relation to weight. In children below 15 kg, the anatomical and physiological differences described above become more important and inhalational apparatus must be adapted, although ketamine can be used without any modifications in technique.

Draw-over anaesthesia for infants

"Adult" breathing systems give rise to problems in small children because the valves have too large a dead space. In addition, vaporizers of the draw-over type do not work effectively at the low minute volumes and flows generated by an infant's lungs. These problems can be overcome in a number of ways.

1. Replace the adult-size breathing valve with an infant-size valve that has a smaller internal volume and dead space. If possible, replace the adult-size SIB with a small bellows or infant resuscitator bag. You must use intubation and controlled ventilation for infants under 10 kg; the flow you generate into the bellows will then be enough to allow the vaporizer to work reasonably accurately.

2. If oxygen is available, you can convert your draw-over system to a continuous-flow mode, either with a Farman entrainer (see Fig. 7.10, page 69) or by connecting a flow of oxygen (or oxygen plus nitrous oxide) to the side-arm of your oxygen-enrichment T-piece and closing off the open end, for example with a bung (Fig. 13.2). You should set the fresh gas flow to 300 ml/kg of body weight per minute with a minimum of 3 litres/min. Intubate and ventilate the patient or allow spontaneous breathing using an Ayre's T-piece system, as described below.

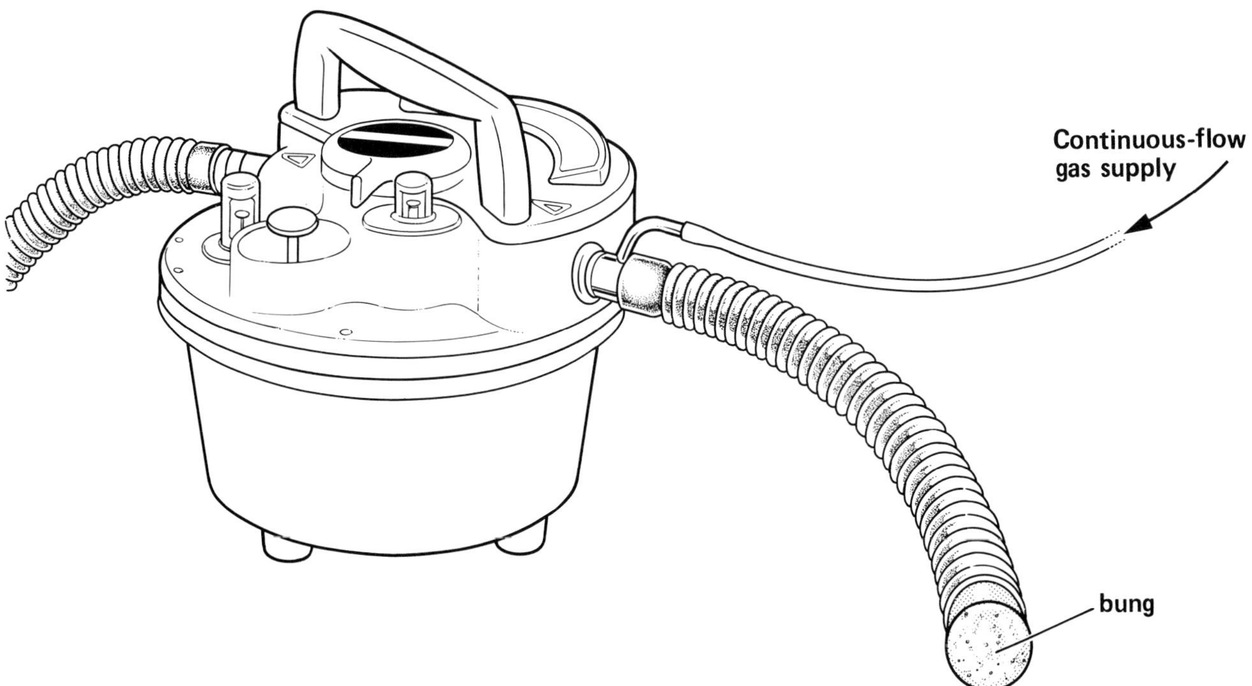

Fig. 13.2. Conversion of draw-over to continuous-flow apparatus.

Continuous-flow anaesthesia for infants

Use a T-piece system (Ayre's T-piece) instead of the Magill breathing system usually used for adults. The valveless T-piece system requires a relatively high gas flow, but is suitable for both spontaneous and controlled ventilation. Spontaneous breathing can be monitored by watching the slight movement of the open-ended reservoir bag. To change to controlled ventilation, hold the bag in your hand with your thumb towards the patient, partly occlude the outlet by curling your little finger round it (this needs practice), and squeeze the bag in the palm of your hand to inflate the lungs (Fig. 13.3). Then release the bag to allow the expired gas to escape.

Monitoring paediatric patients

Continuous monitoring of heart rate and respiration is essential in small children, and a precordial or oesophageal stethoscope is invaluable for this. Use an infant-sized cuff to measure the blood pressure. Palpate the arterial pulses and check the colour and perfusion of the extremities. Monitor the urine flow if a urinary catheter is in place; a good urine output is reassuring. At the end of the operation, check the rectal temperature to ensure that the patient has not become hypothermic.

Anaesthesia during pregnancy and for operative delivery

Physiological changes of pregnancy

Several changes occurring in pregnancy are relevant to anaesthesia. Fairly early in pregnancy the blood volume begins to rise, as does the cardiac output. The increase in plasma volume is not matched by an equivalent increase in the number of red cells, so the haemoglobin concentration falls. As the uterus enlarges, respiration comes to depend more on thoracic than diaphragmatic movement. Gastric emptying becomes less efficient, and a woman who needs anaesthesia in the later stages of pregnancy must therefore always be regarded as having a full stomach. The uterus presses back on the inferior vena cava when the patient lies on her back and this causes a fall in cardiac output. There may also be a severe fall in blood pressure — the "supine hypotension syndrome" — but most

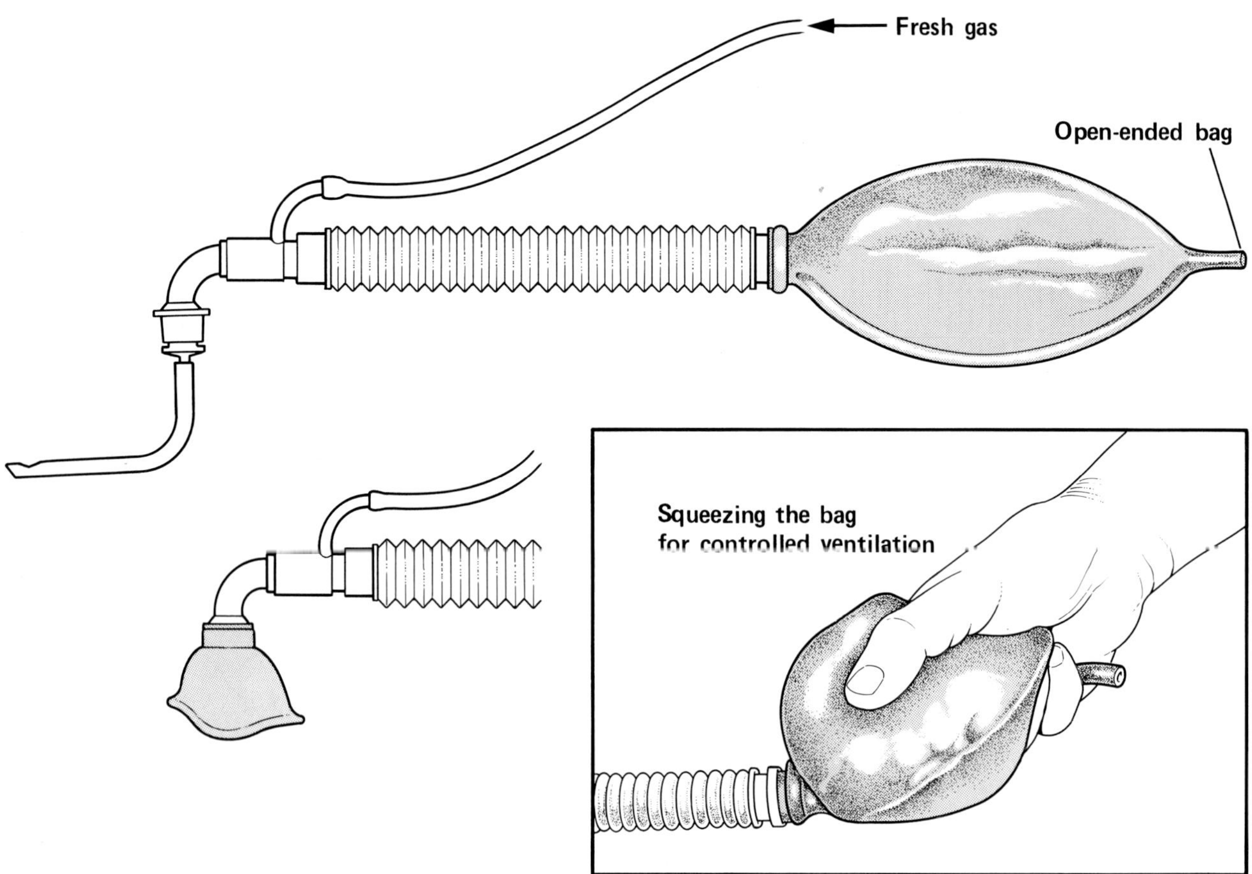

Fig. 13.3. The T-piece breathing system for infants.

non-anaesthetized patients are able to maintain their blood pressure by widespread vasoconstriction. During general or spinal anaesthesia, however, the capacity for vasoconstriction is lost; this is likely to result in a severe fall in blood pressure to levels dangerous for both mother and baby. The condition of supine hypotension can be prevented merely by ensuring that the mother is never fully supine. A pillow or sandbag must always be placed under one hip to tilt the uterus slightly to one side; this is perfectly simple to do even with the patient in the lithotomy position.

Anaesthesia for operative delivery at term

When you anaesthetize a pregnant woman for delivery, remember that you have two patients to deal with: mother and child. Most drugs cross the placenta quickly. This is a problem, since the aim is to anaesthetize the mother, but to allow the baby to be born without any drug-induced depression of body functions, especially of respiration. For this reason, drugs that can cause depression of the fetus, such as sedative premedication, should not be given. Gallamine also crosses the placenta, and its use should be avoided before the umbilical cord is clamped. If a muscle relaxant is necessary, either use another non-depolarizing relaxant drug if available or give increments of suxamethonium.

General anaesthesia for operative delivery

A suitable general anaesthetic technique for operative delivery (caesarean, forceps-assisted, or vacuum extraction) is outlined below.

1. Before inducing anaesthesia give a dose of a liquid antacid, such as sodium citrate 0.3 mol/litre (77.4 g/litre), to neutralize excess gastric acid. Insert a wedge or cushion under one hip to tilt the uterus off the inferior vena cava. *Never* induce anaesthesia with the patient in the lithotomy position. If she is already in that position, her legs must be lowered for induction to avoid regurgitation of gastric contents.

2. Set up a fast-flowing infusion of an appropriate fluid into a large vein and pre-oxygenate the patient.

3. Induce anaesthesia as for an emergency (see page 76): after pre-oxygenation apply cricoid pressure, administer a previously calculated dose of thiopental or ketamine, intubate the patient after giving suxamethonium, and give IPPV with a muscle relaxant. In a pregnant woman at term, intubation is sometimes a little difficult.

4. Do not use high concentrations of ether or halothane, as these will reduce the uterine tone and increase bleeding. Ether 4–5% is safe and will provide sufficient anaesthesia, even in a patient who has received no premedication. If you are using nitrous oxide and oxygen, you may give opiates intravenously once the umbical cord is clamped.

5. Be prepared to give an oxytocic drug (ergometrine or oxytocin) intravenously when requested by the surgeon, but never give ergometrine to a woman with pre-eclampsia.

6. The average blood loss from caesarean section is 600–700 ml, so make sure that you give enough fluid replacement. You may well need to transfuse blood.

7. In addition to looking after the mother, you may have to resuscitate the baby, so be prepared with infant resuscitation equipment and a separate oxygen supply (for more details, see page 114.) If mother and child are both critically ill, it is your clear duty to attend to the mother first. *Always* try to have a trained assistant with you for these cases.

8. At the end of anaesthesia, remember that the mother still has a full stomach; remove the endotracheal tube with her in the lateral position.

Spinal anaesthesia for operative delivery

Low forceps delivery

A low spinal anaesthetic or "saddle block" is ideal for this. Set up an intravenous infusion of an appropriate fluid and inject 1 ml of heavy lidocaine with the patient supported in the sitting position. There is then little risk of hypotension; nevertheless, a wedge should still be used to keep the patient's pelvis tilted when she is put into the lithotomy position, and her blood pressure should be checked every 2 min for at least 10 min.

Caesarean section and internal version

For these procedures a higher block, up to the level of about the tenth thoracic vertebra, is needed. Pre-load the patient with 500–1000 ml of physiological saline, Hartmann's solution, or plasma expander before your lumbar puncture. Inject about 1.5 ml of 5% heavy lidocaine with the patient in the lateral position, and turn her into the horizontal position immediately after injection, but with the pelvis wedged as described above. Be extra vigilant, and actively treat any fall in systolic blood pressure to below 90 mmHg (12.0 kPa), as hypotension can harm both fetus and mother. Always give oxygen to the mother during the operation. Postspinal headache can be a problem, as the mother will need to sit up to nurse the baby, so ensure continuing good hydration for the mother postoperatively.

Anaesthesia for ruptured ectopic pregnancy

The patient will often be a young woman who may be desperately ill with unrecordable blood pressure. Speed is vital. Set up an intravenous infusion of an appropriate fluid using any available large vein — even the femoral vein if necessary. After pre-oxygenation, a rapid induction of anaesthesia with ketamine and suxamethonium is recommended, proceeding to intubation and controlled ventilation with 3% ether in oxygen.

Put in several more intravenous lines as soon as you can; the surgeon may be able to put a catheter temporarily into a pelvic vein for rapid transfusion. In suitable cases, the blood from the abdomen can be filtered and reinfused into the patient (autotransfusion).

Resuscitation of the newborn infant

In a small hospital, you as the anaesthetist may have the added responsibility of immediate care of the newborn baby, especially after an operative delivery. In these circumstances, you must check before anaesthetizing the mother that the necessary neonatal resuscitation equipment is available (Table 5 & Fig. 13.4).

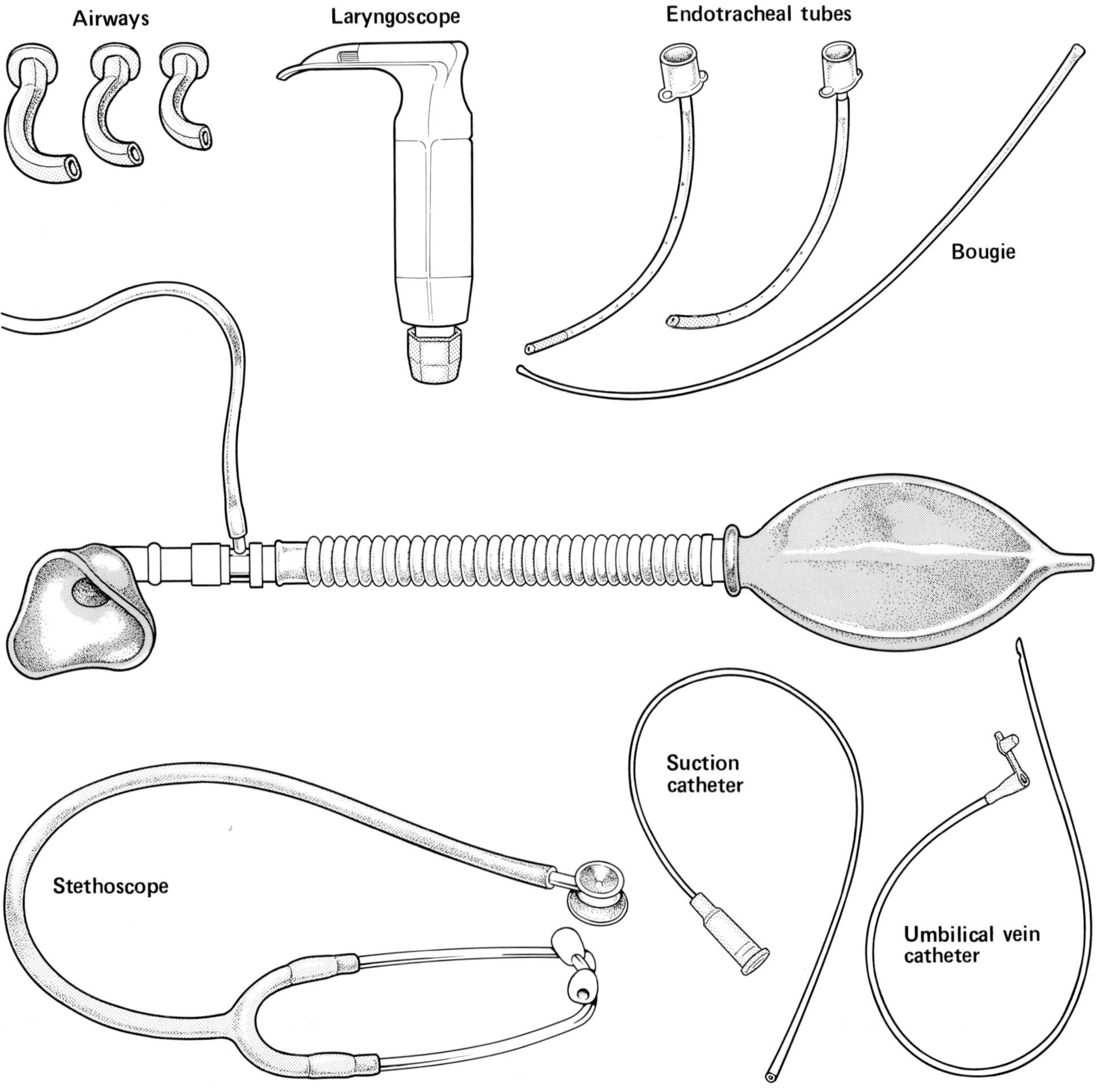

Fig. 13.4. Some of the apparatus needed for neonatal resuscitation.

Table 5. Essential equipment for neonatal resuscitation

Suction apparatus and catheters	Umbilical vein catheter
Laryngoscope	Fluids: plasma expander, 10% glucose
Endotracheal tubes size 2.5 and 3.0 mm and a small bougie/introducer	Drugs: sodium bicarbonate, epinephrine 0.1 mg/ml (1:10 000)
Masks and airways	Oxygen
T-piece circuit *or* paediatric resuscitator bag *or* bellows with oxygen reservoir	

Initial assessment

Many babies require a short period of resuscitation after a difficult birth. Keep the baby warm and gently suck out secretions from the nose and mouth. Immediately assess the heart rate, respiration, and "central" colour (by looking at the lips).

At one minute

If the heart rate is greater than 100 per minute, but respiration is poor, give 100% oxygen and if necessary give a few positive pressure breaths using the T-piece circuit (or paediatric resuscitator bag), mask, and airway.

If the heart rate is less than 60 per minute and respiration is poor, intubate the baby and ventilate the lungs with oxygen. If intubation is difficult (allow only two attempts), use the T-piece circuit to ventilate with a mask and airway. If in any doubt, use mouth-to-mouth/nose resuscitation.

If the heart rate is less than 50 per minute, an assistant should begin cardiac massage.

At five minutes

Most babies respond rapidly to resuscitation. If the heart rate remains less than 60 per minute despite apparently adequate respiration, consider whether the cause is:

- incorrect intubation
- severe birth trauma
- diaphragmatic hernia
- severe blood loss
- hydrops fetalis
- pneumothorax.

Continue resuscitation and insert the catheter into the umbilical vein. Give sodium bicarbonate (diluted in saline) at 2 mmol/kg of body weight, 10 ml of 10% glucose, and 0.2 ml/kg of body weight of 1:10 000 epinephrine.

Specific problems

1. Meconium aspiration: mild cases can be treated by sucking out the fluid from the nose and mouth. A nasogastric tube should be used to empty the stomach. If obvious aspiration has occurred, intubate the trachea and gently suck out the meconium, but do not ventilate. In severe cases the baby may develop respiratory distress, requiring oxygen and antibiotics.

2. Apnoea: prenatal causes of apnoea include intrauterine infection and the administration of narcotics to the mother; postnatal causes include nasal obstruction (which can be overcome with an oral airway) or applying excessive suction to the baby's pharynx.

3. Blood loss can occur as a result of caesarean section, placenta praevia, breech delivery, or twin-to-twin transfusion. The baby will be pale with a tachycardia. Give a plasma substitute or group O Rh-negative blood at 10–30 ml/kg of body weight via an umbilical vein catheter, and repeat this as necessary. The pulse rate should gradually fall to normal.

4. Growth-retarded babies are susceptible to hypoglycaemia, hypocalcaemia, birth asphyxia, and hypothermia.

14
Important medical conditions for the anaesthetist

Anaemia

Severe anaemia interferes with the body's oxygen transport system by reducing the amount of oxygen that can be carried by the blood as oxyhaemoglobin. This means that, to supply the tissues with adequate amounts of oxygen, the heart must pump more blood — hence the tachycardia, flow murmurs, and heart failure sometimes found in anaemic patients. If such a patient is to be subjected to surgery, which may cause blood loss, and to anaesthesia, which may interfere with oxygen transport by the blood, all possible steps must be taken to correct severe anaemia preoperatively. If time is limited, it may only be possible to do this by transfusion.

There is no absolute haemoglobin concentration below which a patient is "unfit for anaesthesia". The decision to anaesthetize a patient depends on the circumstances and the urgency of the need for surgery. Ideally, of course, every patient should have a haemoglobin level "normal" for the community from which he or she comes, but a patient with a ruptured ectopic pregnancy cannot be sent away with iron tablets or even wait for a preoperative blood transfusion. As a rough guide, most anaesthetists prefer not to anaesthetize a patient whose haemoglobin level is below 80 g/litre (5 mmol/litre) if the need for surgery is not urgent, especially if serious blood loss is expected.

Remember that "anaemia" is not a proper diagnosis and may indicate that the patient has another pathological condition that has so far gone undetected — perhaps sickle-cell disease or chronic gastrointestinal bleeding from hookworm infection or a duodenal ulcer. The cause of "incidental" anaemia may be far more in need of treatment than the condition requiring surgery. It is therefore important to investigate anaemic patients properly and not to regard anaemia as a "nuisance" for anaesthesia or to assume that it is necessarily due to parasitic infection.

If you are presented with an anaemic patient with an urgent need for surgery, how should you proceed? Remember that the oxygen-carrying capacity of the patient's blood is lower than normal, so avoid drugs and techniques that may make things worse by lowering the cardiac output (for example deep halothane anaesthesia) or by allowing respiration to become depressed. Ether and ketamine have much in their favour, as they do not depress cardiac output or respiration significantly. Oxygen supplementation is desirable for anaemic patients. Blood lost must be replaced with blood, or the haemoglobin concentration will fall further. Ensure that the patient does not become hypoxic during or after the operation.

Haemoglobinopathies

Haemoglobinopathies are inherited abnormalities of haemoglobin production, which are common in some parts of the world (mostly areas where malaria is prevalent) and in black races. A large number of chemical variants of haemoglobin have been detected, but only a few produce serious disease that may influence anaesthesia; the two most important groups of diseases are the sickling conditions, associated with HbSS, HbAS, and HbSC, and the thalassaemias.

Sickling conditions

Sickle-cell haemoglobin differs from normal adult haemoglobin by a single amino acid in the globin chain, but this small change affects the properties of the molecule so that at low oxygen tensions it forms a crystal (tactoid), which distorts the red cell into an abnormal sickle shape. Sickled cells are rapidly haemolysed, so affected people may suffer from a severe haemolytic anaemia. They also block the capillary microcirculation and trigger thrombosis in vessels. Once started, this process tends to become irreversible and finally results in tissue infarction.

People who carry two genes for sickle-cell haemoglobin (homozygotes, HbSS) have the most serious form of disease, called sickle-cell disease. They are severely anaemic and prone to serious infections, and suffer repeated episodes of arterial thrombosis and pulmonary infarction. The high concentration of HbS in the blood of homozygotes means that sickling is constantly occurring at normal venous oxygen tension, and if they become hypoxic or acidotic it will become even more severe. Homozygotes often die young as a result of repeated infarctions, infections, or sudden aplastic anaemia.

People with a single gene for sickle-cell haemoglobin (heterozygotes, HbAS) have the sickle-cell trait. They are clinically normal, but their red cells are likely to sickle if they become hypoxic or acidotic, when they may develop a severe crisis identical to that of a homozygote. It is therefore important to identify heterozygous patients before anaesthesia and surgery and to ensure that they do not become hypoxic or suffer cardiovascular depression, which could lead to acidosis.

Homozygous patients can often be recognized clinically by their poor growth, by haemolytic anaemia (with sickle cells visible in an ordinary blood film), and by evidence of past infarctions, such as cerebrovascular occlusions and pulmonary and bone infarcts. Heterozygotes can be identified only by laboratory tests; their blood film is usually normal with no sickle cells visible, but the presence of sickle-cell haemoglobin can be detected by incubating the blood with a reducing agent (1% hypochlorite) for an hour, after which sickle cells will be seen. Laboratory tests for detecting sickle-cell haemoglobin rely on its solubility differing from that of normal haemoglobin. For full investigation, haemoglobin electrophoresis is necessary, but this will be possible only at a major referral centre.

A second haemoglobinopathy, found mainly in West Africa, is haemoglobin C disease. Homozygotes (HbCC) suffer from a severe anaemia, but the haemoglobin does not in itself cause sickling. In people who carry one sickle-cell haemoglobin gene and one HbC gene (HbSC) the red cells do have a tendency to sickle, which is intermediate between that seen in people with the HbAS and HbSS genotypes.

It is very important to know preoperatively whether a patient carries sickle-cell haemoglobin. Many patients with sickling crises present with clinical signs resembling those of an acute condition that requires emergency surgery, but such patients do not need an operation. Examples of sickling-associated problems that may be falsely diagnosed are:

- bone infarct mimicking osteomyelitis or septic arthritis
- splenic infarct mimicking an "acute abdomen"
- renal infarct causing haematuria.

Patients with sickling conditions who do need surgery and anaesthesia require special care. A thorough preoperative assessment is essential. Patients with sickle-cell disease will probably already have a multisystem disease, including possible myocardial damage, pulmonary hypertension, and renal failure, and treatment may be needed for these. As anaesthetist, your aim is to prevent the development of hypoxia, acidosis, depressed cardiac output, hypotension, venous stasis, or hypothermia — any of which could trigger the sickling process. Make sure that sufficient fluids are given preoperatively, and in the operating theatre be generous with fluid replacement (but be careful not to overload patients with sickle-cell disease who may have poor cardiac function). The use of ether or ketamine as the main anaesthetic is suggested, since both these agents maintain a good cardiac output. Oxygen supplementation should be used during and after anaesthesia. Avoid heavy doses of opiates, which may cause respiratory depression, and keep the patient warm at all times. Cold produces venous stasis, and the patient's oxygen requirement will go up if shivering starts.

Thalassaemias

These conditions are also inherited abnormalities of haemoglobin production, but in this case, there is a failure to produce one of the normal component globin chains. Instead, fetal or other abnormal haemoglobins, which have abnormal oxygen-binding properties, are produced. Depending on the variety of thalassaemia, there is a more or less severe anaemia, and the patient may be undersized and weak, but sickling is not a problem unless the patient also carries the gene for sickle-cell haemoglobin (sickle-cell thalassaemia).

Glucose-6-phosphate dehydrogenase deficiency

This is an inherited, sex-linked abnormality of red cell metabolism. It is normally asymptomatic, but patients may react with acute severe haemolysis to the stress of acute illness or after the administration of a variety of drugs. The drugs most often implicated include antimalarial drugs, sulfonamides, nitrofurans, analgesics (especially aspirin), *p*-aminosalicylic acid, and chloramphenicol.

Cardiovascular diseases

Patients with cardiac disease present a number of problems if they require anaesthesia. The function of the heart, which may well be abnormal to start with, can be further affected by potent drugs that the patient is receiving, such as β-adrenoceptor blockers, digoxin, or calcium-channel blockers. Added to this are the anxiety and catecholamine release that come with an operation, as well as the cardiovascular depression that is, to a certain extent, an effect of all anaesthetic drugs, both local and general. It is not surprising that problems occur from time to time when such patients are anaesthetized.

Ischaemic heart disease

Patients with ischaemic heart disease who need anaesthesia and surgery have a greater-than-average risk of complications. Narrowed coronary arteries need a higher perfusion pressure than normal to allow blood to perfuse the myocardium. Any degree of hypotension may therefore be harmful, but so may hypertensive crises, which drastically increase the amount of work the left ventricle has to do, even though blood flow through the coronary arteries may be incapable of further increase.

No patient should have elective surgery within 6 months of a myocardial infarction; there is a substantial risk of another infarction occurring postoperatively, whether general or conduction anaesthesia is used, and the mortality associated with such infarcts is very high — over 50%. For a patient who requires emergency surgery within 3 months of an infarction, a conduction technique is preferable, with the anaesthetist taking great care to avoid hypotension. A patient with ischaemic heart disease requiring elective surgery should be strongly considered for referral.

Patients with chronic ischaemia (i.e., those with stable angina pectoris, a previous history of myocardial infarction, or evidence of ischaemia on an electrocardiogram but without symptoms) can be given careful anaesthesia (general or conduction) for elective surgery. A careful preoperative assessment is needed, with a search for evidence of poor myocardial function, for example dyspnoea or cardiac failure, and the presence of dysrhythmias. A full, 12-lead electrocardiogram should be obtained, and X-ray examination of the chest should also be routine. Patients who are in a stable condition while taking drugs should not have their treatment altered or stopped. Measurement of the patient's serum potassium concentration is essential, especially if digoxin or a diuretic is being taken. The general principle should be that no patient should have elective surgery if a further preoperative improvement in condition is possible.

If general anaesthesia is chosen, a technique based on intubation and relaxant with IPPV is preferable to deep inhalational anaesthesia, which may cause severe myocardial depression. In many patients with ischaemic heart disease, laryngoscopy can provoke a severe tachycardia and dysrhythmias, and many anaesthetists prefer to give an intravenous bolus of lidocaine (1 mg/kg of body weight) about 30 s before laryngoscopy in an attempt to prevent this. During anaesthesia, try to avoid sudden swings in blood pressure, and maintain good oxygenation and ventilation (hence the recommendation for IPPV). Good postoperative analgesia is important, as severe pain can cause hypertension and dysrhythmias. If you have access to an electrocardiograph with a continuous display, use it from before induction of anaesthesia until full recovery; if you have only a paper-writing electrocardiograph, you should connect the electrodes to the patient, so that if any clinical signs make you suspect dysrhythmia during the operation, you can make a rapid diagnosis from a rhythm strip.

Myocardial diseases (cardiomyopathies)

These conditions are characterized by damage to myocardial tissue, which may affect muscular performance, electrical activity, or both. The causes may be nutritional (for example beriberi, alcoholism), congenital (fibroelastosis, muscular dystrophy), infective (Chagas' disease), or idiopathic. Most of these conditions present with progressive cardiac dilatation and cardiac failure. Anaesthesia and surgery are then extremely hazardous and, in all but the direst emergency, such patients should be referred for a full cardiac assessment. If anaesthesia is unavoidable, consider the use of a field or nerve block, combined with ketamine if necessary. General and spinal anaesthetics, unless given by an experienced specialist anaesthetist, are best avoided.

Valvular heart disease

Patients with valvular heart disease have impaired cardiac function. You must assess from a medical history and an examination how severe the patient's disease is. This requires careful inquiry about the patient's symptoms and exercise tolerance. A patient with mitral valve disease with mild symptoms only will normally withstand anaesthesia well, but severe dyspnoea or cardiac failure points to severe disease and the need for referral. Unfortunately, the management of patients with aortic valvular disease is not so straightforward; these patients may develop symptoms only in the preterminal phase of their disease. They should certainly not have elective anaesthesia if there is any hint of angina, effort syncope, or blackouts or if there is any clinical, electrocardiographic, or radiographic evidence of left ventricular hypertrophy. For emergencies, use low spinal anaesthesia (taking steps to avoid hypotension) or a nerve/field block as the technique of choice. If general anaesthesia is unavoidable, do not use thiopental, which can cause fatal cardiovascular collapse.

A potential problem in patients with valvular disease is that they may develop bacterial endocarditis as a result of transient bacteraemia from instrumentation in the mouth or other parts of the body, for example the urinary tract. Antibacterial prophylaxis is therefore essential. A high level of antibiotic is required only for the peri-operative period, and for most purposes this can be achieved by penicillin and streptomycin.[1]

Hypertension

Elective anaesthesia and surgery are contraindicated in any patient with sustained hypertension and blood pressure greater than 180 mmHg (24.0 kPa) systolic or 110 mmHg (14.7 kPa) diastolic. This degree of hypertension will be associated with clinical signs of left ventricular hypertrophy on chest radiographs and electrocardiograms, retinal abnormality, and possibly renal damage. In an emergency, the same principles apply to the management of a hypertensive patient as to a patient who has had a recent myocardial infarction. Consider a conduction anaesthetic technique and make every attempt to avoid hypotension, which can precipitate a cerebrovascular accident or myocardial infarction. Severely hypertensive patients whose need for surgery is not urgent should be referred.

Patients whose hypertension has been reasonably well controlled can safely be anaesthetized. It is important not to discontinue any regular treatment with antihypertensive drugs, or the patient's blood pressure may go out of control. After a full assessment of the patient, including obtaining a chest radiograph and an electrocardiogram and measuring serum electrolyte concentrations (especially if the patient is taking diuretic drugs), you may carefully use any suitable anaesthetic technique, with the exception of ketamine, which tends to raise the blood pressure. If the patient is receiving treatment with β-adrenoceptor blockers, the treatment should be continued, but remember that the patient will be unable to compensate for blood loss with a tachycardia, so special attention is needed.

Respiratory diseases

Tuberculosis

Tuberculosis is a multisystem disease whose respiratory and other effects may present problems for the anaesthetist. There are firstly the problems of anaesthetizing a patient with a severe systemic illness, who may have nutritional problems and abnormal fluid losses from fever combined with a poor oral intake of fluid and water, and a high metabolic rate requiring a greater supply of oxygen than normal.

Local problems in the lung — the production of sputum, chronic cough, and haemoptysis — may lead to segmental or lobar collapse and hence to inadequate ventilation and oxygenation. Endotracheal tubes may quickly become blocked with secretions, so frequent suction may be necessary. In sick patients who

[1] For an adult, crystalline benzylpenicillin (600 mg, 1 million IU) mixed with procaine benzylpenicillin (600 mg, 600 000 IU) should be given intramuscularly with streptomycin (1 g) 30–60 min before surgery. Phenoxymethylpenicillin (500 mg) should be given by mouth or intramuscularly 6 hours later.

cannot cough effectively, a nasotracheal tube may be left in place after surgery or a tracheostomy performed to allow for aspiration of secretions.

Contamination of anaesthetic equipment with infected secretions must also be considered. If you have to anaesthetize a patient with tuberculosis, use either a disposable endotracheal tube, which you can then throw away, or a red rubber tube which, after thorough cleaning with soap and water, can be autoclaved. The patient's breathing valve and anaesthetic tubing will also need to be sterilized. Most valves (except all-metal Heidbrink valves) will tolerate only chemical sterilization. Black, antistatic breathing hose can be autoclaved. It is unlikely that the SIB in a draw-over system will be contaminated, but if you sterilize an SIB be careful, as many of these are damaged by autoclaving. If you use a Magill breathing system on a Boyle's machine, the whole system should be autoclaved, as the patient can breathe directly into the bag. If you cannot see how to overcome contamination problems with inhalational anaesthesia, use ketamine or a conduction or spinal technique instead.

Asthma

For elective anaesthesia and surgery in a patient with a history of asthma, the asthmatic condition should be under control and the patient should have had no recent infections or severe wheezing attacks. If the patient takes drugs regularly, treatment must not be discontinued. Special inquiry must be made about any former use of steroids, systemically or by inhaler. Any patient who has formerly been admitted to hospital for an asthmatic attack should be referred for assessment. Conduction anaesthesia combined with intravenous sedation with small doses of diazepam may be a better choice of technique than conduction anaesthesia alone or general anaesthesia.

If general anaesthesia is necessary, premedication with an antihistamine such as promethazine together with 100 mg of hydrocortisone is advisable. It is important to avoid laryngoscopy and intubation during light anaesthesia, as this is very likely to lead to severe bronchospasm. Ketamine is quite suitable for intravenous induction because of its bronchodilator properties. For short procedures, it is advisable to use a face-mask technique after induction and avoid intubation altogether. Use an oxygen concentration of 30% or more in the inspired gas. If intubation is required, deepen the anaesthesia with an inhalational agent and intubate without giving a relaxant. A patient anaesthetized deeply enough to allow laryngoscopy is unlikely to develop bronchospasm as a result of intubation. Ether and halothane are both good bronchodilators, but ether has the advantage that, should bronchospasm develop, epinephrine (0.5 mg subcutaneously) can safely be given (this would be very dangerous with halothane or trichloroethylene since these anaesthetics sensitize the heart to the dysrhythmic effects of catecholamines). Aminophylline (up to 250 mg for an adult by slow intravenous injection) can be used as an alternative to epinephrine if bronchospasm develops; it is compatible with any inhalational agent.

At the end of any procedure that includes endotracheal intubation, extubate with the patient in the lateral position and still deeply anaesthetized; otherwise the laryngeal stimulation might again provoke intense bronchospasm.

Chronic bronchitis

The patient with chronic bronchitis has some degree of irreversible airway obstruction. In taking a history, you should ask about exercise tolerance, smoking, and sputum production. The patient must be told to give up cigarettes completely at least 2 weeks before the operation. Simple clinical tests of lung function may be valuable; healthy people can blow out a lighted match 20 cm from the mouth without pursing their lips and can count aloud in a normal voice from 1 to 40 without pausing to draw breath. The nature of the operation is of great importance; elective surgery on the upper abdomen is contraindicated, since respiratory failure in the postoperative period is likely. Patients needing such surgery must be referred to a hospital where their lungs can be ventilated artificially for 1–2 days postoperatively if necessary.

For emergency surgery, use a technique with intubation and IPPV with added oxygen. Postoperatively, give oxygen at not more than 1 litre/min via a nasal catheter. Be careful with opiates, as the patient may be unusually sensitive to respiratory depression. For upper abdominal analgesia, consider repeated intercostal blocks. With 0.5% bupivacaine these blocks can last 6–8 hours, during which time the patient can breathe and cough up sputum without pain. The patient should of course receive regular chest physiotherapy both preoperatively and postoperatively.

Diabetes

The diabetic patient who needs elective surgery is not difficult to handle. In the short term, the only major theoretical risk is that undetected hypoglycaemia might occur during anaesthesia. In fact most general anaesthetics, including ether, halothane, and ketamine, cause a small and harmless rise in the blood sugar concentration and are therefore safe to use. (There is a widespread, but unfounded belief that diabetic patients should not be given ether.) Thiopental and nitrous oxide have little effect on the blood sugar concentration; no anaesthetic causes it to fall.

Diabetic patients can be classified according to whether their diabetes is controlled with insulin (insulin-dependent diabetes) or by diet and/or oral hypoglycaemic drugs (non-insulin-dependent diabetes). If the patient's diabetes is controlled by diet alone, you can normally use an unmodified standard anaesthetic technique suitable for the patient's condition and the nature of the operation.

For insulin-dependent patients, ensure that the diabetes is under reasonably good control. On the morning of the operation, do not give the patient food or insulin; this will ensure a normal or slightly elevated blood sugar concentration, which will tend to rise slowly. Measure the blood sugar concentration shortly before anaesthesia. It will probably be 7–12 mmol/litre, but if it is higher than 12 mmol/litre, give 2–4 International Units of soluble insulin intravenously or subcutaneously and measure it again in an hour. Give further doses of insulin as necessary. As an alternative, if frequent blood sugar measurements are impossible, put 8 International Units of soluble insulin into 500 ml of 5% glucose and infuse intravenously at 100 ml/hour for a normal-sized adult. Continue with this regimen until the patient can eat again and then return to normal antidiabetic treatment. This scheme is simple and will maintain blood glucose levels in most diabetic patients in the range 5–14 mmol/litre; however, regular checks of blood glucose concentration should be made and the regimen changed if necessary. Note that, if glass infusion bottles are used, the dose of insulin will need to be increased by about 30%, as the glass adsorbs insulin. Where several patients are due to undergo surgery on a given day, diabetic patients should be first on the list, since this makes the timing and control of their insulin regimen much easier.

Patients with non-insulin-dependent diabetes controlled with oral hypoglycaemic drugs should not take their drugs on the morning of anaesthesia. Because certain drugs, notably chlorpropamide, have a very long duration of action, there is some risk of hypoglycaemia, so the blood sugar concentration should be checked every few hours until the patient is able to eat again. If difficulties arise with these patients, it may be simpler to switch them temporarily to control with insulin, using the glucose-plus-insulin infusion regimen described above.

Emergency surgery

The diabetic patient requiring emergency surgery is rather different. If the patient's diabetes is out of control, there is danger from both diabetes and the condition requiring surgery. The patient may well have severe volume depletion, acidosis, hyperglycaemia, severe potassium depletion, hyperosmolality, and acute gastric dilatation. In these circumstances, medical resuscitation usually has priority over surgical need, since any kind of anaesthesia attempted before correction of the metabolic upset could prove rapidly fatal. Resuscitation will require large volumes of saline with potassium supplementation (under careful laboratory control). There is no point in giving much more than 4 International Units of insulin per hour, but levels must be maintained either by hourly intramuscular injections or by continuous intravenous infusion. The patient will need a nasogastric tube and a urinary catheter. If the need for surgery is urgent, a conduction anaesthetic technique can be used once the circulating volume has been fully restored. Before a general anaesthetic can be given, the potassium deficit and acidosis must also have been corrected, or life-threatening dysrhythmias are likely. The level of blood sugar is much less important; it is better left on the high side of normal.

Obesity

Obese patients (who may also be diabetic) face a number of problems when anaesthesia is necessary. Obesity is often associated with hypertension — though with a very fat arm the blood pressure is difficult to measure and may appear high when in fact it is not. Because of the extra body mass, the cardiac output must be greater than in a non-obese person; more work is also required during exertion, which places greater stress on the heart. The association of smoking, obesity, and hypertension is often a fatal one with or without anaesthesia. Because of the mass of fat in the abdomen, diaphragmatic breathing is impaired and the chest wall may also be abnormally rigid because of fatty infiltration. Breathing becomes even more inefficient when the patient is lying down, so IPPV during anaesthesia is recommended, with oxygen enrichment if possible.

Extra technical problems are found in obese patients. The fat neck makes airway control and intubation difficult, and excess subcutaneous fat leads to difficulty with venepuncture and conduction anaesthesia. Do not give drugs on a weight basis, as this will result in an overdose. For most drugs given intravenously, a 120 kg patient needs only about 130% of the normal dose for an adult of 60–70 kg. For general anaesthesia in the obese patient, a technique based on endotracheal intubation with IPPV using relaxants is recommended.

Malnutrition

Malnourished patients require special care and should ideally be allowed a period of intensive feeding (beginning gradually) before surgery to enable them to survive the metabolic demands of surgery and then be capable of the process of healing.

Multiple deficiencies may be present in malnutrition. Iron, folate, and vitamin B-12 deficiencies are likely. An initial measurement of haemoglobin concentration may be misleadingly high as a result of dehydration. Other vitamin deficiencies, for example beriberi, may give rise to muscle weakness with consequent respiratory or cardiac failure. Liver function is likely to be depressed, with low levels of enzyme activity resulting in an increased duration of the action of many drugs. Low plasma protein levels mean that oedema, either peripheral or pulmonary, can easily develop in response to what seems a minor fluid overload. If surgery is absolutely necessary in such a malnourished patient, it is probably safer to avoid general anaesthesia and use whatever conduction technique is likely to cause the least physiological disturbance.

Chronic renal failure

Patients with renal failure may be suffering from a variety of related medical problems, including diabetes, anaemia, electrolyte disturbances, hypertension, and chronic acidosis. The anaesthetist needs to pay particular attention to the drugs used during anaesthesia, as those normally excreted by the kidney will have an abnormally marked and prolonged action. Problems are most likely to arise with the prolonged action of non-depolarizing relaxants. Gallamine in particular is totally dependent on renal excretion and should never be used in a patient with renal failure. Opiates also depend on the kidney for excretion, so must be used with caution. If the haemoglobin concentration is low it is important to maintain a good cardiac output. For anything but a minor procedure, a urinary catheter should be inserted to monitor urinary output, and a good diuresis should be maintained.

15
Supplies and equipment

Gas supplies

Oxygen

Oxygen is valuable and sometimes essential during anaesthesia, and it is important to have a sufficient and reliable source of supply. Fortunately, oxygen is widely available, since it is needed for a variety of industrial applications. The principle of manufacture of industrial oxygen is identical to that of medical oxygen, i.e., the fractional distillation of air, so chemical impurities are unlikely in either form, and industrial oxygen is perfectly safe for medical use. It may also be easier to obtain and less expensive. If you obtain oxygen from an unorthodox source, you must be certain that the cylinder, especially if it is not standard, does indeed contain oxygen, so take a few breaths yourself. If there is no smell and you do not feel dizzy, the gas must be oxygen or air. Determine which by dropping a lighted match into a jar full of the gas (*but turn off the supply of gas and move well away from the cylinder first*).

The oxygen supply from the cylinder must be connected to the anaesthetic apparatus through a suitable pressure-reducing valve. For larger cylinders this valve is incorporated into the cylinder pressure gauge; on a Boyle's machine both the gauge and reducing valve are part of the machine. When connecting cylinders to anaesthetic apparatus, be sure that the connectors are free from dust or foreign bodies that might cause the valves to stick. Never apply grease or oil, as it could catch fire in pure oxygen, especially at high pressure. Remember that the contents of an oxygen cylinder are in compressed gaseous form and that the reading on the cylinder pressure gauge will therefore fall proportionately as the cylinder contents are used. A full oxygen cylinder normally has a pressure of around 13 400 kPa (132 atmospheres, 2000 p.s.i.). It should always be replaced if the pressure within is less than 800 kPa (8 atmospheres, 120 p.s.i.) as failure is then imminent.

Oxygen concentrators

These devices have recently been developed for medical use. They are capable of producing gas containing a high concentration of oxygen (> 90%) at a clinically useful flow rate (3–4 litres/min) by physical separation of oxygen from air. The Dräger Permox and similar concentrator units have a compressor from which filtered air is pumped alternately through two tanks containing a molecular sieve (zeolite) that allows oxygen to pass, but retains nitrogen (Fig. 15.1). When the zeolite in one tank is saturated with nitrogen, the flow is automatically switched to the other tank while the first is purged. The unit needs only a supply of electricity to provide oxygen and may be the solution to logistic problems of oxygen supply. At the moment the units produced need regular servicing; there may be problems in humid climates; and an oxygen monitor to check the output would be desirable to reassure the clinician. However, there is great potential for these units, especially in remote hospitals. In addition to the small unit described, which is suitable for anaesthesia, a larger installation is also available, which could supply the oxygen requirements of an entire hospital.

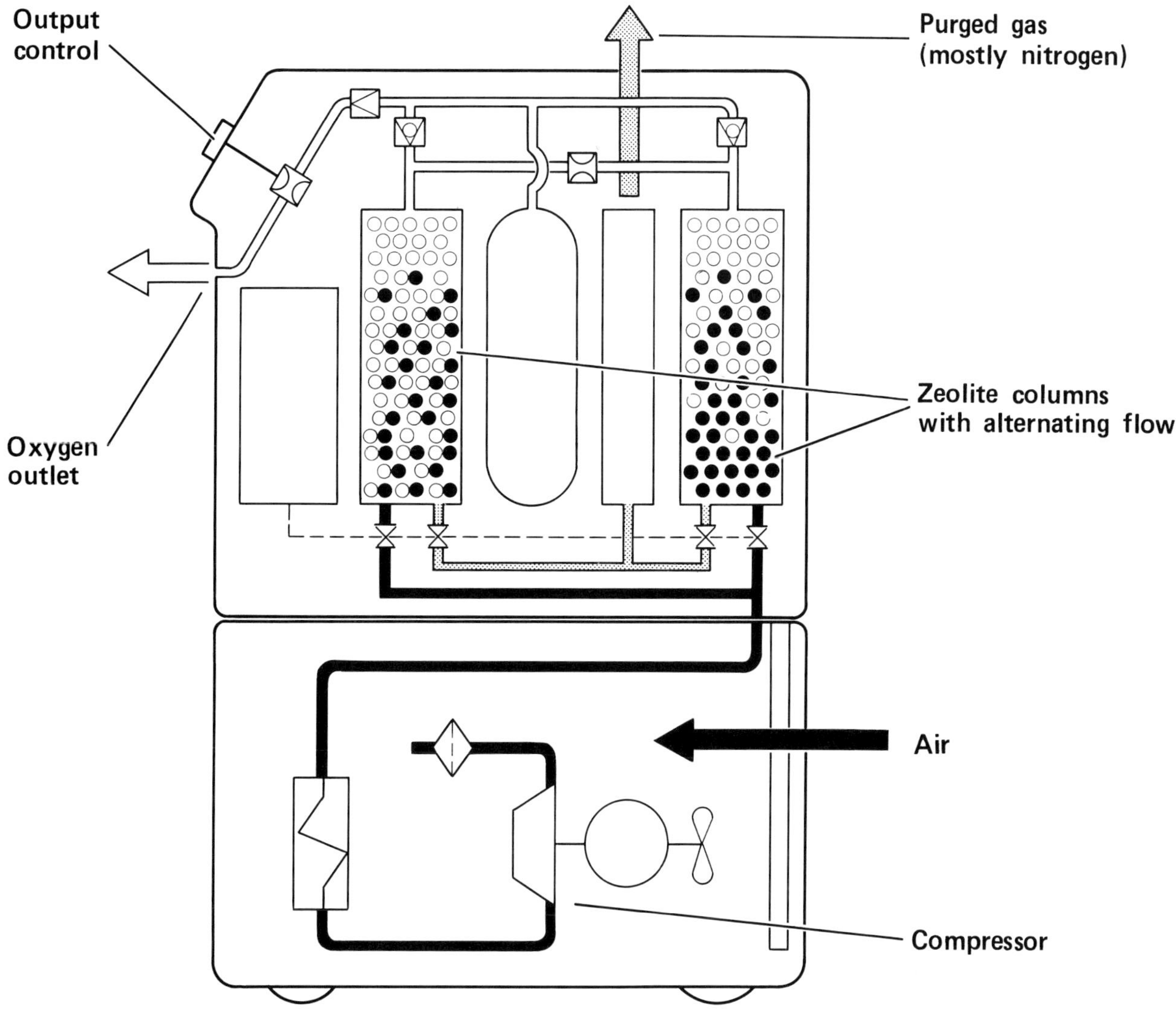

Fig. 15.1. Oxygen concentrator.

Nitrous oxide

Nitrous oxide was one of the first agents to be used as an inhalational anaesthetic, but it is now rarely given alone because of its low potency. When given in combination with other anaesthetics, however, nitrous oxide has the advantage of reducing the amount of the other agents needed to achieve the required level of anaesthesia. Full nitrous oxide cylinders have a pressure of 5200 kPa (51 atmospheres, 750 p.s.i.), but since the cylinder contents are mostly liquid, this pressure is maintained until the cylinder is about 85% used, after which the pressure falls rapidly.

Drugs

A minimum list of essential drugs is given in the WHO Model List of Essential Drugs (see WHO Technical Report Series, No. 722, 1985). This list is regularly reviewed and updated.[1] For the drugs mentioned in this handbook, see Annex 4.

[1] A new list will be published in the WHO Technical Report Series in 1988.

Anaesthetic equipment

The anaesthetic equipment listed below represents the minimum that a district hospital should possess.

Anaesthetic face masks	• 2 of each size, infant to large adult; total 14
Oropharyngeal airways	• 2 of each size 00 to 5; total 12
Laryngoscopes	• 2 handles + 3 pairs of blades, or 4 plastic laryngoscopes (2 adult + 2 paediatric) • 12 spare bulbs + 30 batteries (or 8 rechargeable batteries + charger)
Endotracheal tubes	• sizes 2.5–10 mm (internal diameter) in 0.5 mm steps, Oxford or Magill or similar, with cuffs only on sizes > 6 mm
Urethral bougies	• for use as intubating stylets
Magill's intubating forceps	• in an emergency, ovum forceps can be used instead
Endotracheal tube connectors	• 15 mm plastic (can be connected directly to the breathing valve), 3 for each tube size
Catheter mounts (sometimes also called endotracheal tube connectors)	• antistatic rubber, 4
Breathing hose and connectors	• 2 lengths of 1 metre antistatic tubing • 4 lengths of 30 cm tubing for connection of vaporizers • T-piece for oxygen enrichment
Breathing valves	• universal non-rebreathing valves (6 adult + 2 paediatric)
Breathing systems (for continuous-flow anaesthesia)	• Ayre's T-piece system • Magill breathing system
Self-inflating bellows or bag (SIB)	• 1 for adults + 1 for children
Anaesthetic vaporizers (draw-over type)	• for ether, halothane, and trichloroethylene
Equipment for intravenous use	• needles and cannulas, including paediatric sizes and an umbilical vein catheter • infusion sets
Spinal needles	• range of sizes, 18-gauge to 25-gauge
Suction apparatus	

Suction apparatus

A reliable sucker is essential and must be available for any general or conduction anaesthetic procedure. A large variety of suction apparatus is available, powered by electricity, by compressed gas, or by hand/foot (Fig. 15.2). Electrical suckers are most convenient to use, provided there is not a power cut. Mechanically operated suckers are a good back-up, both for electrical failures and for use on patients in transit. They can be operated by pedal or by pressing a trigger. Suckers

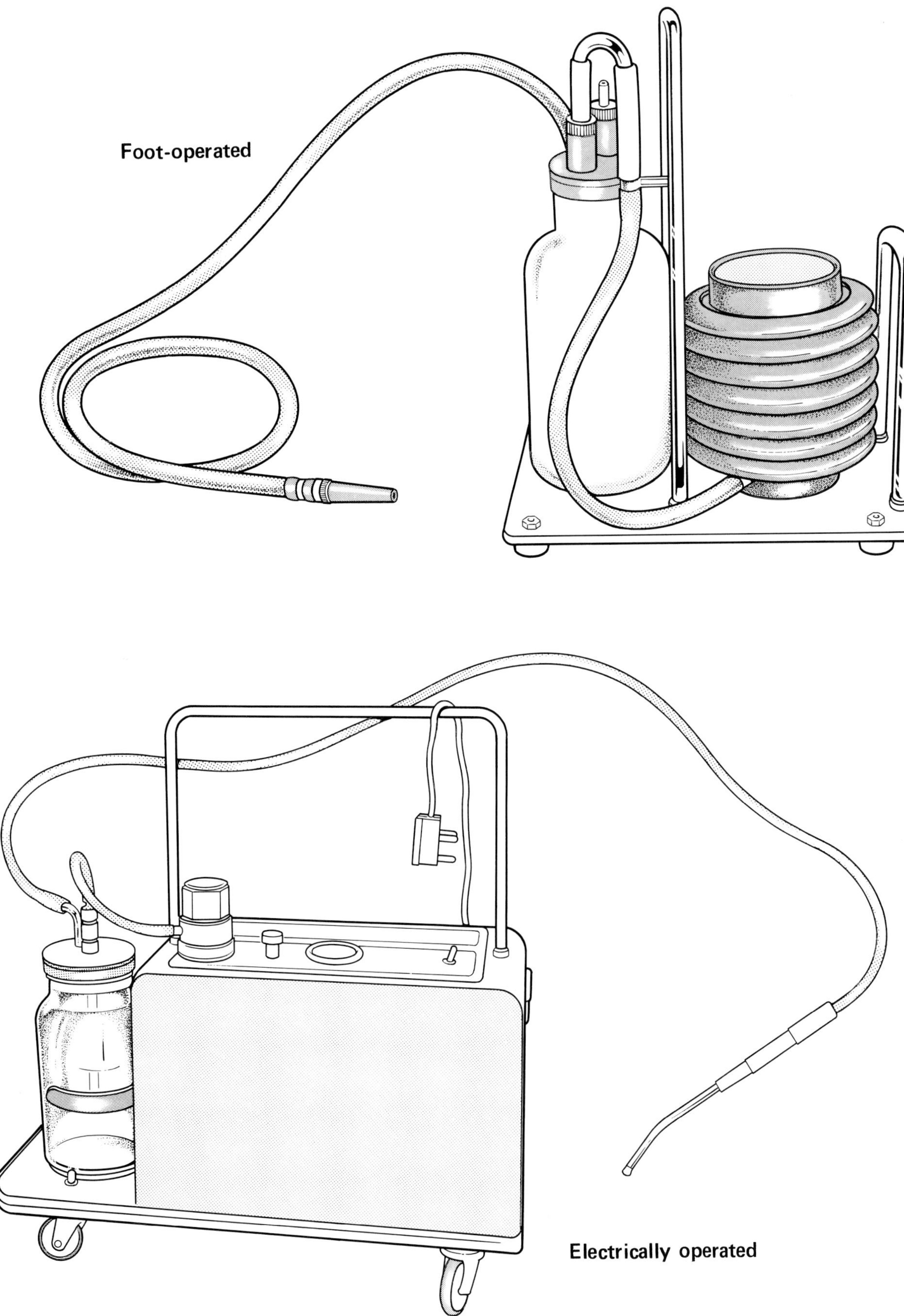

Fig. 15.2. Suction apparatus.

powered by compressed gas are efficient, but not advisable for hospitals where gas supplies may be limited and oxygen is best reserved for breathing. Non-medical compressed air, if available, can serve as a power source.

Test your sucker regularly. A good test is to see how long it takes to deal with 100 ml of thick soup (or equivalent). This will give you an idea of how efficient the sucker will be when used in a patient's pharynx in an emergency.

Storage and maintenance of equipment

You must have a detailed inventory listing all the equipment you possess. Anticipate the need for further supplies of items such as batteries, bulbs, and tubes, and order replacements well in advance. Allow at least 6 months for anything that needs to be imported. Check all your apparatus at least once a month. It should be stored in a cool, dry place (for example a lockable cupboard). Put bungs in any open-ended vaporizers to keep out dust and insects, and join breathing hoses end-to-end in a circle. Wipe down your apparatus regularly with a dilute, soapy antiseptic solution. If your vaporizers are to be unused for a week or more, drain off the anaesthetic agents (but not the water). Drain all vaporizers at least once a month to remove debris and antioxidants contained in the anaesthetic formulations, to avoid parts of the vaporizer becoming stuck.

Check your equipment regularly for leaks, both by inspecting it and by pressurizing it (do this by hand for an SIB by squeezing the bag or bellows after putting a bung in the valve).

Establish contact with your national referral hospital for the servicing of equipment. Many draw-over vaporizers are relatively simple to service and do not need to be sent back to the manufacturer. Do not attempt to service vaporizers yourself unless you have been fully trained to do so and are equipped with a complete set of spares and a service manual.

After each anaesthetic procedure, pieces of apparatus that have been in contact with the patient (for example laryngoscope blade, face mask, airway, endotracheal tube) should be thoroughly scrubbed with soapy, warm water and allowed to dry in a dust-free place. Formal sterilization of these items is not necessary in most cases. After use on infected patients, however, apparatus should be cleaned as above and then all-metal or metal and rubber items autoclaved, for example metal laryngoscope blade (without the bulb) and rubber airway; other items should be sterilized chemically, with reference to the manufacturer's instructions.

Annex 1

Check-list for draw-over anaesthetic apparatus

Keep a copy of this list by your anaesthetic apparatus. You must fully check all apparatus before beginning anaesthesia.

Oxygen cylinder and flow meter

Turn on supply of gas from cylinder, and check pressure and flow. Also check spare cylinder.

Oxygen reservoir

Check for proper assembly of T-piece, and make sure that air inlet is unobstructed.

Vaporizer

Check that the vaporizer is filled (using only stocks of anaesthetic in their original containers). Check that connections fit, and set dials to zero.

Self-inflating bag/bellows

Check connections and, if applicable, position of magnet on bellows.

Breathing and connecting hoses

Check connections and correct assembly of breathing system (see Fig. 7.7, page 65).

Breathing valve

Test the valve yourself and check it visually; the bobbin or valve leaflets should move during breathing.

Check for leaks

Squeeze the bag or bellows while using your hand to block the connector that joins the breathing valve to the patient. No air should escape.

Make sure that you have:

- face mask of suitable size
- oropharyngeal airway of suitable size
- tested laryngoscope and spare
- endotracheal tube of suitable size (test cuff by inflating)
- tested suction apparatus
- table or trolley that can be tilted head-down
- all drugs you may need.

NEVER INDUCE ANAESTHESIA UNLESS AN ASSISTANT IS PRESENT.

Annex 2

Check-list for continuous-flow (Boyle's) anaesthetic apparatus

Keep a copy of this list by your anaesthetic apparatus. You must fully check all apparatus before beginning anaesthesia.

Emergency equipment

You *must* have a suitable resuscitation device, for example a self-inflating bag or bellows, to ventilate the lungs of the patient in case your gas supply fails.

Oxygen supplies

For machines fitted with cylinder-only supply

Turn on the oxygen supply from the cylinder in use and check the pressure. Turn on the supply from the reserve cylinder, check the pressure, and turn it off again. Check that you have a third cylinder available to replace the cylinder in use when it is exhausted.

For machines fitted with a piped gas supply

Check the source of your piped gas supply. Check that you have a full cylinder of oxygen fitted to your machine in case the piped supply fails.

All machines

Turn off all gas supplies except one oxygen cylinder or piped supply. Open *all* rotameters. Oxygen should flow through only one rotameter tube (the oxygen one!). *If this does not happen, do not use the machine.*

If your machine has an oxygen-failure warning device, test it as follows:

> Turn on the gas supply from one oxygen cylinder (pipeline disconnected if fitted) and one nitrous oxide cylinder (if fitted).
>
> Open rotameter taps to give a flow of oxygen (and nitrous oxide also if fitted) of 5 litres/min.
>
> Turn off the oxygen supply at the cylinder. If a functioning warning device is fitted, an alarm should sound as the oxygen rotameter bobbin starts to fall (this may take a few seconds). On some machines, oxygen failure automatically cuts off the nitrous oxide supply also.
>
> After the test remember to open the oxygen cylinder valve again.

Avoid using a machine that does not have a functioning oxygen-failure alarm. If you have no alternative, you must record the oxygen cylinder pressure every 5 min throughout anaesthesia and change cylinders when the cylinder pressure drops below 1500 kPa (15 atmospheres, 220 p.s.i.).

You must *never* begin anaesthesia with a machine that has only a single source of oxygen, i.e., only one cylinder or one pipeline.

Nitrous oxide

Check the pressure in the nitrous oxide cylinder in use and in the reserve cylinder. If the pressure in a nitrous oxide cylinder at room temperature is less than 5200 kPa (51 atmospheres, 750 p.s.i.), the cylinder is less than 15% full.

Rotameters

Inspect visually for cracks. Make sure that the bobbins do not stick in the tubes.

Emergency oxygen

Locate and turn on the emergency oxygen (bypass) button or tap. A high flow of oxygen should be delivered from the gas outlet. Note that this supply does not pass through the oxygen rotameter.

Vaporizers

Check that all vaporizers are firmly connected and filled with the correct anaesthetic agent (from stocks of anaesthetic in their original containers). Check that all filling ports are firmly closed, and that concentration dials are set to zero. A Boyle's bottle should have both the lever and the plunger pulled up.

Leaks

Check your machine once a month for leaks (or immediately, if you suspect one) by "painting" suspect areas with soapy water and watching for bubbles.

Breathing system

Check for correct assembly (see Fig. 7.14, page 73).

Make sure that you have:

- face mask of suitable size
- oropharyngeal airway of suitable size
- tested laryngoscope and spare
- endotracheal tube of suitable size (test cuff by inflating)
- tested suction apparatus
- table or trolley that can be tilted head-down
- all drugs you may need.

NEVER INDUCE ANAESTHESIA UNLESS AN ASSISTANT IS PRESENT.

Annex 3
Anaesthesia record

You should keep a record of every anaesthetic that you give. The specimen record chart shown opposite could be combined with a preoperative check-list (see Fig. 5.1, page 48) and a postoperative instruction sheet.

Anaesthesia Record

Date	Age	Weight	BP	Hb g%	Hospital No. ....
					Surname ....
Premedication		Effect			First Name ....
					Ward .... Blood group ....
Anaesthetist		Surgeon			Operation

ANAESTHETIST'S NOTES including: relevant history/clinical findings/drugs/allergies.

ANAESTHETIC TECHNIQUE

TIME		DRUG	Total Dose
Chart each dose as given	1		
	2		
	3		
	4		
	5		
	6		

°C		EVENTS
40	300	
35	250	
30	200	
25	150	
	100	
	80	
	60	
	40	
	30	REMARKS
	20	
	10	
	0	

I.V. fluids	Blood loss

Annex 4
Drugs used in anaesthesia

Alcuronium
Aluminium hydroxide
Atropine
Bupivacaine
Calcium gluconate
Chloral hydrate
Diazepam
Epinephrine
Ether
Gallamine
Halothane
Ketamine
Lidocaine
Methohexital
Morphine
Nalorphine
Naloxone
Neostigmine
Nitrous oxide
Pentobarbital
Pethidine
Prilocaine
Promethazine
Sodium bicarbonate
Sodium citrate
Thiopental
Trichloroethylene

Names and addresses of local suppliers and agents

(List any useful local addresses here.)

Index